CHRONIC PAIN:

Taking Command

of Our Healing!

Understanding the emotional trauma underlying Chronic Pain

BY

WM. R.B. ANDERSON, Ph.D.

with

JESSE F. TAYLOR, Ph.D.

Published by
NEW ENERGY PRESS
1225 LaSalle Suite1604
Minneapolis, MN 55403

Cover by Hansen Gjerness Advertising
Illustrations by Paul Michael Davies and Brian Hansen
First Edition:1995

Library of Congress Cataloging-in-Publication Data

Anderson, Wm. R. B., date

Chronic pain: taking command of our healing!
:understanding the emotional trauma underlying chronic pain/by Wm. R.B. Anderson
with Jesse F. Taylor, date, - 1st ed.

p. cm--

ISBN 0-9642979-0-6

1. Chronic pain--Psychosomatic aspects. 2. Chronic
pain-- Alternative treatment. 3. Psychic trauma
I. Taylor, Jesse F.

RB127.A53 1994   94-37679
616',0472--dc20   CIP

Note

The ideas and information presented herein are not intended to supplant successful, on-going treatments but rather, to enhance them.

PART ONE

PART TWO

ACKNOWLEDGMENTS

To Barbara Brennan, her staff, and my classmates at the Barbara Brennan Healing School for the thorough grounding in healing principles.

To Char Peterson for her valuable contribution and to Earl Joseph, Petra Henttonen, Peg Keller, Malcolm Rosholt and Margaret Smith for their reading of the manuscript and their useful comments.

To Paul Michael Davies, Brian Hansen, Dave Gjerness, and Gary Hansen for their advice and artistic contributions.

To Pat Bell, Jim Luker, and our editor, Margaret Young, for their advice and assistance in bringing the book to publication.

To those staff members at Sister Kenny Institute who have provided support in this endeavor.

To my wife, Kate Brennan Anderson, my mother, Betty Jean Anderson, and my children, Tom, Tim, Sasha, and Paul for their love, support and contributions.

Dedication
To the clients in my private practice and at the
Sister Kenny Institute, who have been my
greatest teachers.

Forword

I first met Bill Anderson in Fort Collins, Colorado at a meeting of The International Association for New Science. He was presenting a paper from his doctoral dissertation on Chronic Pain. At that time he was just beginning his exploration of alternative healing techniques. I was impressed by his enthusiasm for the subject as well as his natural acceptance of intuitive insights. He and I spent many hours discussing not only the ideas introduced in the conference but the path he had followed to arrive at his own ideas. As we both lived in the same city, those discussions continued well after the conference was over. As Bill became clearer in his own understanding of the healing process, the ideas for the book emerged. This volume is the distillation of those ideas.

In some ways, we are an unlikely pair of collaborators. I, some twenty-five years older, have a "left-brain" orientation and have spent my life in traditional academic disciplines.

Bill, on the other hand, has a distinctly "right brain" orientation and arrived at the more traditional academic pursuits via an unusual route which led through a career in professional hockey coupled with a lengthy study of Eastern mysticism.

Bill's deeply intuitive approach to life is fascinating to me. His understanding and acceptance of any idea is heavily dependent on his personal experience with that idea. He has an inherent suspicion of abstract and theoretical proposals.

My background is from the other end of the continuum. The training I received led me always to discount intuitive insights and to search for hard data. It is only in the last few years that I have come to see how limiting that view is.

I mention this because I suspect that there will be a number of readers whose paradigm of health treatment has been limited, as was mine, to the view that mainstream medical practice is the only plausible alternative.

Our confidence in mainstream medical practice is based on an assumption that most medical procedures have been "proven" through scientific studies. The reality is that while many procedures have been tested in the laboratory and pronounced effective, a great deal of practice has emerged as a result of trial and error. This in no way denigrates the practice of medicine but it lets us see the practice of medicine without "white coat and test-tube" image that seems to elevate doctors to a level beyond mere mortals.

Medical doctors, like the rest of us, do what works. When they are confronted with a patient who needs help, they call on their experience and training to make a decision. Sometimes they select a treatment which has been tested in laboratories and in double-blind studies and proven to be effective. At other times they select a treatment that, in their experience, has worked a high proportion of the time. This does not make them quacks. They are "practicing" medicine. Their experience and training is what makes them expert in their field. That training and experience has its limits. Their training is based on a set of theories about how the body works but the problem is that this understanding of the body and the healing process is not complete.

Unfortunately, the Medical Establishment is slow to expand its range of theories in the search for effective treatments. For example, while many doctors will, informally, admit that emotional effects are important in healing, they are hesitant to give professional credence to procedures which treat emotions in order to heal physical illness. "Psychosomatic" symptoms, that is, physical symptoms that are thought to be caused by the mind rather than a physical problem, are frequently dismissed by physicians as something over which they have no control. While this should be evidence that there is a connection between physical and mental states, traditional medicine has ignored it as "imagined illness." *Placebo effects*, which will be discussed later, provide additional examples of the relationship between mind and body. Too often, emotional or psychological effects are ignored because they are not in the healing paradigm of the doctor.

Happily, this is changing. Mainstream medicine is now beginning to expand its paradigms. More attention is being paid to the relationship of the mind and the physical body. As this field develops, testing procedures will emerge to make the mind-body connections.

Beginning with Norman Cousins, who wrote of the healing power of laughter in *The Anatomy of an Illness*, interest in the mind-body relationship has resulted in a growing number of studies of those factors in the healing process which depend not alone on a surgeon's knife and a bottle of pills. An excellent reference work is Richard Gerber's *Vibrational Medicine* which provides excellent background in theory, history, and spiritual philosophy of these approaches to healing. More recently, Bill Moyer's television series *Healing and the Mind*, a season or so ago, brought increased awareness of alternative therapies to mainstream America.

But for those who need "hard data" before allowing themselves to explore alternative approaches, Dr. Daniel J. Benor has provided the most useful work to date.

In *Healing Research - Holistic Energy Medicine and Spirituality*, Dr. Benor reviews and evaluates the scientific research, double blind studies and laboratory studies in language which is accessible to the non-scientist. Anyone looking for the scientific study of alternative healing techniques would do well to search out this book.

Readers will search in vain, however, for such discussions here. It is not our intent to provide scholarly, scientific data, however valuable that may be. Rather, we hope to provide ideas and exercises which have been effective in Bill's work in his private practice as well as his work with chronic pain clients at the Sister Kenny Institute. The basis for the treatments is that emotional trauma lies at the base of most chronic pain. Once that emotional trauma is released, healing can occur. The ideas and treatments have evolved as Bill has begun to understand his own experience and the experience of his clients more clearly. It is an unfolding process and one which requires that both the healer and the client pay attention to their intuition. Each individual has a deep understanding of his or her source of healing. Getting in touch with that source is the key to healing. There are no "one size fits all" treatments here. The reader in search of healing must feel a resonance to one or another idea as it is presented and mold that idea to fit their need. If he or she can do this on a deep intuitive level without left-brain chatter interfering, there is a good chance of success.

From the beginning, this has been Bill's book. As his successful clinic experience and study grew, it became clear that he had something of value to communicate to the countless people who suffer from chronic pain. He is sharing his experience and the intuitional insights which have grown from that experience. My contribution has been to help expand and clarify these insights as they have unfolded in the writing of the book.

These ideas and exercises are offered as possibilities for those people who are searching for something more than their present medical therapy is offering. They are not offered as an alternative to successful therapy but, rather, as an aid to hasten healing. It is a firm tenet in this book that no single therapy is "correct" for a given health problem. We all have a healing process that is unique to ourselves. For most people, emotional trauma has a response in the physical body and we need to search in ourselves to find what that effect is for us. Finding the emotional component that underlies pain is a complicated process when it is analyzed intellectually. It becomes much less complicated when it is understood intuitively

Jesse F. Taylor, Ph.D.

Minneapolis, 1994

Introduction

This book is written for those people who are struggling with chronic pain. For many people, the label of chronic pain is a life sentence of helpless discomfort with no explanation and no relief. Their treatments have involved tests, counseling and medications for the symptoms which continue to demand relief. My experience in working with people with chronic pain has led me to see that there are other alternatives in this struggle and that it is possible to develop a program of self-healing.

By self-healing, I do not mean a mystical trance in which the chronic pain sufferer closes his eyes and wills the pain to be gone from his body in a miraculous instant. What I mean is that through understanding how pain finds its way into our bodies, we can assert our own methods of dealing with it. We are not without power. We need not be victims of pain. But to do this we must accept the fact that our own bodies are unique and that there is no single remedy for illness, disease, or pain. We must accept that our own intuition is able to select the remedy most appropriate to our own body and we must allow our intuition to work for us.

I am not suggesting here, that the medical treatments which are commonly prescribed are wrong. I am saying that as long as they provide relief, they should be continued. But if pain continues, then other methods must be explored. To carry out this exploration and devise those other methods, we need to have a way of understanding pain.

Part One of this book will try to provide a discussion of chronic pain that includes not just the reactions of the pain sensors in our body but also the emotional component that intensifies our experience of pain. This new way of looking at our pain may help us find relief in some surprising ways.

In Part Two, we will develop a plan for our own healing. This will include some self-analysis. As we explore the attitudes we have about our life and our pain, we will examine some profiles of behavior that may be limiting our healing. We will review some exercises in breathing and relaxation which often help reduce the immediate discomfort and allow us to spend more energy in healing. Finally, we will discuss some alternative healing techniqes and look at those aspects of our life that help us to heal and those which seem to prevent us from healing.

This plan will be of our own making and we can adjust it as we move along the path. The important part of this approach is that the plan is unique to each individual. If I have learned anything from my experience it is that each person has unique and individual healing needs and we only learn which ones work for us by our own experience.

Although I have done much academic study and I am continuing to learn about chronic pain and healing methods, I want to stress that what is contained in this book is filtered through my own experience and what the reader takes from this book must be filtered through his or her own experience as well.

Because that experience is so important to the ideas and approaches in this book, it makes sense that the readers should have some idea of the life from which those ideas evolved. What follows is a brief description of my life as I now understand it.

Who is William R. B. Anderson, Ph.D.?

First of all, almost everyone calls me Bill and I like it that way. To an outside observer, my life began as the typical story of "Just Plain Bill" in Mid-America. But like most outside observations, that impression doesn't tell even half the story. The youngest of four children, I was raised in a comfortable suburb with all the usual activities to absorb my life. Like most young boys, sports became an important part of my life.

But "Just Plain Bill" fell in love with being a sports star. In fact, my first experience with pain was as an active young athlete aspiring to become a professional sports figure. I saw pain, at that time, as part of the test I needed to pass to make it in the sports world.

On the outside, I was Cool Hand Luke. I didn't let anything bother me. I was the perfect son of Ward and June Cleaver. I was the perfect athlete who played in spite of any pain or injury.

Although I did not realize it, I had begun to use pain to fill a need. Playing while injured seemed heroic to me in those days and I arranged my life in that illusion. For many years, I by-passed the pain and injury to stay in the game. Through high school and college sports, and, finally, in professional hockey, I saw the pain and injury I experienced as a badge of honor, a testimony that I didn't "give up." But the energy I gave to controlling that pain and ignoring the effects on my body finally took it's toll. My body had finally had enough of the "heroism" I had believed in for so long and I was confronted with the grim reality of a body which no longer withstood the strains I unthinkingly demanded. I had to give up the dream.

But, looking back, I realize now that even that "grim reality" was a dream too! I had only switched from being the "hero" to being the "victim." I seemed to understand my life only through labels society had taught me.

My sports career was terminated and, at the same time, my personal life and the thriving business I had started began to falter. I was faced with financial ruin and a broken marriage. Unable to understand my own potential, I saw myself as a victim of events and the actions of others. That victim status served me as an escape. When I felt unable to find a resolution to a difficult business problem, I took refuge in the pain resulting from a car accident to avoid confronting what had to be done. My pain helped me delay facing the unpleasant choices I eventually had to make.

It took me a long time to realize that the Bill Anderson I thought I was, had never existed! My challenge now was to find the "real" Bill Anderson.

I returned to school — this time to study, not to play hockey. Stimulated by the courses in psychology as well as an interest in Eastern philosophy, I began to see myself as part of an unfolding reality.

For my doctoral dissertation, I worked with chronic pain patients in a study that examined the relationship of pain to emotions. As I began to understand how that relationship worked for me, I found I could help patients make the same connection.

The study of these behavior patterns, made it clear that what contributed to my own pain and suffering was the holding back of my inner longings. It was the denial of my anger, guilt, abuse, and sexuality that lay hidden deep within the cells of my body. It has been my own pain that has led me, reluctantly, to explore and discover my inner truth.

I also discovered that there were needs which were satisfied through my vulnerability as a victim. I used my pain to extract attention and love from those around me. As a victim, I received attention that I felt I, otherwise, would not have deserved.

When this realization crystallized, it was the beginning of my life's work. I now devote myself to helping people become aware of the nature of their pain and how inner trauma keeps them from realizing their true selves.

My present view is that all our experience is connected. We cannot isolate and treat only a physical pain, a suppressed emotion or a psychological condition. All these things must be healed together. And the healing begins within us. Delivering our body to someone else to be repaired, whether it be a medical doctor or a psychologist, will only heal one small part of our life. Those specialists can help us, but what matters most is what we do for ourselves. We must take command of our own healing.

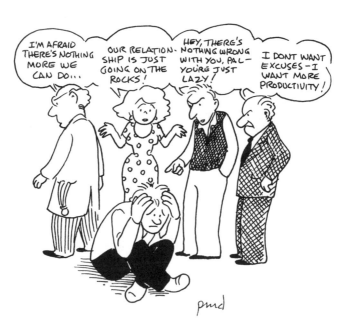

- 1 -

Our Pain and the Healing Process

Pain has become a large part of our everyday vocabulary. Those of us with chronic pain go to one medical professional after another to seek relief from the relentless discomfort. Often we are accumulating only bills and an impressive vocabulary. Then the day arrives when the clinician tells us that there is nothing more to be done for the pain!

We find ourselves in a no-win situation. We have had our pain so long that family, friends, and co-workers are beginning to question and doubt if such pain really exists. It begins to dawn on us that we are alone with our pain. No one is listening any more. Fear of a lonely future of perpetual pain begins to form. Our job security, our income, as well as our physical well-being, is in jeopardy. Our relationships are suffering and we know people are tired of hearing about our problems.

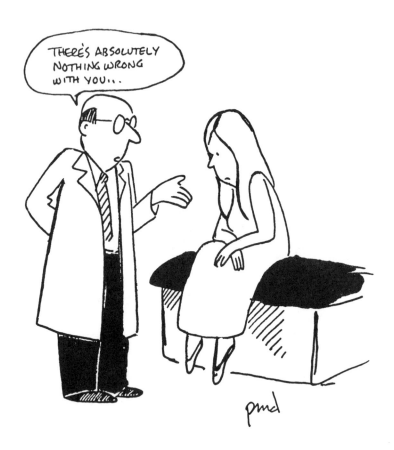

Since there seems to be no one to turn to for help, it is not surprising that suicide often becomes a consideration.

We feel powerless as we confront our inability to explain the trauma of a pain with no foreseeable end and no clear explanation. We are gripped by an irrational fear that this sinister force will take over our lives.

Our first step toward healing is to conquer this fear! We must put our pain in perspective. There is no question that the pain is real, but we must recognize that it is a different kind of pain than the acute pain we have often experienced.

As painful as a toothache is, we are not frightened by it because we know that certain steps can be taken to end the pain. We need only to get through the night until the dentist's office opens. We experiment with our favorite pain killers and wait. Our experience with chronic pain, however, is very different.

Our trips to the doctor have not stopped the pain. As time goes on, the medications seem to become a permanent part of our daily routine. Nothing changes. The doctors have said that they can find no reason for the pain. They cannot tell us how long we will have this pain and we begin to wonder if they think we are imagining it.

Because our experience with acute pain creates an over-simplified image of how pain develops, we wrongly conclude that if a specialist can't find a treatment that it is either "all in our mind" or that there is nothing that can be done. We will see that, though it is not *all in the mind*, it is, in one sense, *all in the brain*.

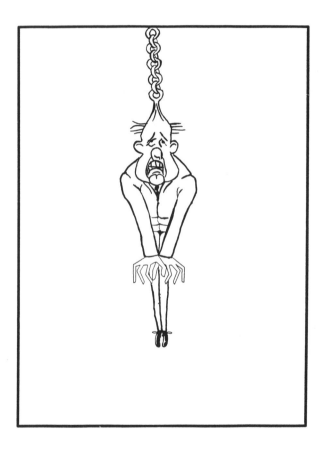

"The chain of pain lies mainly in the brain...

What do we know about pain?

One point about pain that we don't consider very much is that the pain and the injured part of the body are two different things. A physical injury is an event in which the cells of the body are being stressed in some way. A bruise appears on the the shin when it is hit by some hard object. The cells are reacting to this stress. The pain does not reflect this activity, it is simply the message sent to brain about the stressed cells in the shin. It is "experienced" in the brain but we "feel" it in the shin.

When we talk about our pain, we have some general terms that we use. Our head "aches," we have a "sore knee," or we have "hurt" our finger. These words are very general. When we try to be more specific, we use analogies. We compare pain to something that we can see. It is "as sharp as a knife," or "stabs like a sword." Sometimes we compare it to the "throbbing" sensation of the heart or it can be a "burning" pain.

Whether the experience is a result of a finger on a hot iron or on a cool marble, the pain receptors send the message. To describe the experience, our mind finds a comparison, an analogy, to help us talk about it or understand it. It is through the use of these analogies that most of us think about pain. The analogies become the *reality* of pain for us. But there are other ways to understand pain.

Western science, for example, tries to understand pain by studying the way sensations of pain are sent to the brain. They have traced the pain impulses through the nerve endings in the skin, muscles and some organs of the body and followed these nerve connections through the spinal cord to the brain. They have concluded that these messages are the sensations of pain with which we are familiar. They are understood to be warnings that there is some problem in the body.

In our everyday "non-science" life, we ignore the idea that there are *pain receptors* which are communicating messages to the brain. We rub the injured knee because our brain tells us there is a problem there. Sometimes that even reduces the pain by distracting the pain receptors which now have to send messages about this new event that is occurring on the knee.

Probably the best example of the difference between pain and a physical injury itself, is the the problem of *referred pain*. There are parts of the body which do not have pain receptors. When those parts of the body are injured, the message is sent from pain receptors located in the same section of the body but which are not necessarily injured. For example, the heart has no pain receptors so the pain from a heart attack is "felt" not in the heart, but rather in the arm, the neck, or the shoulders.

Western medicine thinks of pain as the *messages* sent to the brain. They go to the part of the body which has sent the message to see what is wrong. They think of pain as a fire alarm system.

When something destructive occurs someplace in the body, a message is sent to the brain. The pain we experience is the fire alarm. This triggers a variety of behaviors which the brain initiates to correct the problem. These behaviors may be as obvious as moving the fingers away from the hot stove or as subtle as releasing white cells to control infections or endorphins to dull pain. In this sense, our pain is an important security device that protects us from disasters.

But when the problem is going to be a prolonged one, as in an operation or a dental filling, we recognize that the pain is no longer needed as an alarm system so we try to shut off the alarm by providing an anesthetic. We take an aspirin for a headache and in extreme cases, when there seems to be no other way of shutting off the alarm system, surgery is used to disconnect the nerves from the brain so no more messages can be sent.

The body, itself, sometimes fails to send the alarm messages. Most of us have had experiences in which we were involved in a very intense experience, in a sports competition, for example, in which our attention was so focused on what we were doing that we failed to notice that we had bruised our shin. Only later when the excitement was over, did our brain get the message that there was a problem in the shin.

In recent years, surgery, use of electrical impulses in such devices as the Transcutaneous Electrical Nerve Stimulator (TENS) units, massage therapy, chiropractic treatments, as well as guided imagery and energy therapy have been increasingly common in the treatment of pain. When we are thinking about the treatment of pain from the point of view of medicine as it is practiced in the Western world, we think of these techniques as intervening to stop the pain messages. We do not think of them as "curing" the injury or illness. We are only "disabling the alarm system."

But the Western model of medicine is not the only way of thinking about healing. To use another analogy, it is only one kind of map. It shows us certain parts of the terrain. There are other maps which show us other parts of the terrain that may also be useful. For example, a map that shows all the highways can give us an idea of what cities we will travel through and how long it will take. A map that shows the elevations that we will be traveling through gives us another picture of our trip altogether. This is important in thinking about pain and what we can do about it. If we use only one kind of map, we are limited in the information we have. It is helpful, therefore, to consider what other maps are available.

Eastern medicine, for example, provides us with a different kind of "map." They see the body as a system of *meridians* and *chakras* through which a vital force of energy flows in the body. This life force is called *Chi* or *Prana* and illness is presumed to be a problem of blocked or unbalanced life force.

The Eastern healer works primarily to balance or unblock this flow of energy. Acupuncture and breathing exercises such as Qi Gong are techniques which are used to bring about healing. This model "maps" the body, not as a bundle of complicated circuits, but rather as channels of energy flowing through and permeating all the cells of the body. This system of health treatment has been used for thousands of years in the Far East and is still used today along with Western medical techniques. In the West, our medical practice has been slow to experiment with these techniques although acupuncture is becoming much more common in many clinics in this country.

So we have at least two ways of thinking about the body and about pain. In the Western model, the emphasis is on finding a way to heal the tissue or bone, or to kill the virus, or bacteria which is attacking healthy cells. Drugs and surgery are the most frequent tools of the Western doctor. Most of us reared in the Western tradition tend to believe that the only way we can be healed is to go to the doctor to be repaired in much the same way we take our cars to the garage to be repaired. When there appears to be no treatment or drug, we are at a loss to know how to proceed. We are left with the diagnosis of Chronic Pain and a search for more and better pain killers.

Eastern medicine, on the other hand, looks for ways to affect the flow of healing energy. Acupuncture needles, herbs, breathing techniques and meditation all play a part in their healing process. These too, are not a hundred per cent effective. But both Eastern and Western models can claim dramatic healing triumphs.

Faith healing, Native American shamanism, and aboriginal techniques provide yet another way of looking at illness. In these cases, spirits are assumed to play some part in the healing process. These, too, have had some amazing healing records. So the list of possible healing models grows and we have more and more to choose from in developing a healing plan.

It is interesting to note that in most healing approaches, many of the treatments are intended to encourage the body to activate its own healing mechanisms. Drugs are used to stimulate the immune system, or an acupuncture needle tries to remove a blockage in the energy flow.

As patients, we often overlook the possibility that our body is healing itself because we are distracted by the elaborate and skilled procedures which are being used as catalysts for our body's own healing.

The idea of the body healing itself is not all that strange, after all. Most of us have paid little or no attention to a cut finger once we have stopped the flow of blood. The skin heals up and the whole incident is forgotten. A cold often clears up, untreated, after six or seven days. But when the pain becomes too great, we turn to others for help. We leap to the conclusion that if the body could heal the problem it would have done so already. But we may be too hasty in that assumption.

Research on the *placebo effect* suggests that there is more to be learned about the effect of the belief system on the body's ability to heal itself. When scientists are testing the effectiveness of a drug, for example, they give the drug they expect to be beneficial to a certain number of patients and give a substance that has no potential for healing such as a sugar pill to another group of patients suffering from the same problem. This is called a *placebo*. Frequently, however, some of those people who were treated with the placebo recover as well as those treated with the authentic drug. Occasionally this effect is explained by saying that those patients who were healed with the placebo didn't really have the ailment anyway. More careful scientists simply say that, based on the available evidence, they cannot explain the phenomenon. But, if pressed, a frequent explanation for this unexpected outcome is that the patient's belief in the drug was so strong that the healing process was triggered even though there was no drug administered.

Until recently, this effect was largely ignored by the scientific community because they had no way to explain it. Their belief system did not include a body which could heal itself. But since the evidence continues to pile up and there are more and more cases of healing which cannot be explained, the possibilities are being taken more seriously.

Those of us with chronic pain problems should not dismiss the possibility that we can create a "miracle" ourselves.

Another aspect of pain which offers some important help for people with chronic pain is that of the relationship of emotion to pain. None of us doubt that emotions can effect the bodily functions in some way. We know about the effect of stress on the blood pressure, for example. We are at least vaguely aware of how depression seems to make us vulnerable to colds and virus infections. We have all had a "stress headache" at one time or another. But we may not have become as conscious of how positive emotions seem to decrease pain. Norman Cousin's book, *Anatomy of an Illness,* as we have noted before, describes how he used laughter to eliminate the effects of a very debilitating disease. We should not rule out that possibility in our own life.

But there is more to the emotional component than simply thinking positively. The possibility that emotional trauma is an underlying factor in our pain should not be dismissed. If we go back to the idea that pain is an impression in the brain, the connection between the emotional intensity of an experience and the intensity of the pain which we feel is not difficult to make. What we need, however, is a way of thinking about that connection because none of the medical models we have discussed emphasize it. Let me suggest an approach that will include emotional trauma as a possibility.

Let us assume that our bodies are filled with the life force or energy which the Eastern philosophies discuss. Even if we don't understand all the philosophy behind it, we can still see that there is a difference between matter which is alive and matter which is dead. That "aliveness" can be thought of as a life force or energy. And when something is alive it is "conscious." That is, it is aware of itself and the environment around it. Our cells have their own awareness. Not only do they have the *pain receptors* which send the message to the brain, they also have the vital energy which flows through them supporting the healthy life. But those cells can also be affected by emotions. The effect of stress on the body is well known. Emotions are the stress carriers. So as emotional trauma sweeps through the body, it leaves the effect or "memory" of that trauma in the cells. If this "memory" is not released, the vital healing energy is distorted by the trauma and that distortion is translated as pain by the receptors which send the messages to the brain.

So what I am suggesting is this. Let us suppose that as a child, I had a very traumatic experience. Let us say I was sexually molested, for example. The emotional trauma of that experience would have flooded through my body and the stressed cells would have been distorted. Now, because the experience was so horrible, I might have blocked it from my conscious mind. The stressed cells are still there with their "memory." At some point another traumatic experience occurs. I am in a car accident, for example. That emotional trauma floods through my body as well. But this time, because I do not block the awareness, the cells, already stressed, start the pain receptors jangling. Once they are started, they continue to send the alarm messages well after the physical damage of the car accident has been repaired reflecting the stress of the sexual molestation which is still there. Only after that stress has been released will the alarm messages stop.

Thinking about illness or pain in this way leads us to a different perspective on treatment of the problem. As in Eastern medicine we are no longer looking for a treatment of the symptoms through medications or surgery but are searching for a way to release the blockage itself. Particularly in the case of chronic pain, the source of this blockage can be intimately tied to negative emotions, thoughts, and feelings.

These emotions affect the life force which is carried throughout the body in the oxygen that nourishes the cells, nerves, arteries, veins, and muscles. This means that our thoughts, emotions, and feelings are directly affecting the cells and the nervous system even though we are unaware of it at a conscious level.

The relationship of physical pain and emotional trauma is beginning to receive attention by all branches of the healing community. More and more cancer programs include an examination of emotional stresses that may be related to the disease itself. Psycho-immune diseases such as arthritis, fibromyalgia, and chronic fatigue syndrome appear to be related to the emotions.

As we begin the task of uncovering the possible emotional trauma that lies below our pain, we can call upon both the traditional and non-traditional methods in our search. We must take back the responsibility for our healing and use both the health care and healing communities for the services that they provide best. But we must begin with our own plan so that we know what we need and we can organize our healing plan to serve us.

Part One of this book is intended to present a discussion of various aspects of chronic pain which people with may want to consider as they analyze their own situation. Part Two begins with a suggestion that a journal is helpful in discovering how chronic pain is related to the full range of our everyday life. Our pain is not simply a physical ailment which is isolated from the rest of our life. To prepare for writing this journal, I will present a few questions at the end of each chapter which readers may wish to ponder in regard to their own situations. There are no right answers and you cannot fail the test. Just let your mind and feelings play around the ideas.

Questions for consideration:

◆ *If I had to draw a map of my pain, what would it include?*

An Alarm System?

Meridians?

A Life Force or Energy?

Energy blocked by emotional Trauma?

◆ *How is my map limiting my possibilities?*

- 2 -

An Overview of Pain

Pain can enter our lives and change forever the life we have been living. Until that happens, we may spend very little time thinking about pain. But when it comes, it absorbs all our attention. We experience pain's potential for both fire and ice. To help us make sense of the experience, it is helpful to develop a concept of the nature of pain and its underlying causes.

As has been discussed, pain can be defined as the body's feedback system, an indicator of something wrong. There are two types of pain, *acute* and *chronic*. *Acute pain* is any physical pain that is short in duration and has a discernible cause. It warns us that something is wrong and we may need to take action. It is the pain that has helped us survive our younger years. Acute pain is the sharp stabbing pain we feel when we step on a rock with our bare feet. It is the injection of a needle filled with Novocaine puncturing the skin at the dentist office. It may represent some type of warning for us to take immediate action. When we feel this pain, we move away from the hot fire or we decide to seek medical treatment for the severe pain caused by an injury or illness.

Chronic pain is usually defined by the medical community as a pain that lasts well over the normal recovery time expected from an injury. Such pain usually lasts six months or more. This extended pain experience often carries with it psychological problems which complicate recovery. The experience of one of my client's, serves as an example.

One day, hurrying from the office, Bob fell down a flight of stairs. Although he felt shaken and suffered a few minor bumps and bruises, he didn't think much about the accident. In fact, he didn't even report the incident to the person in charge of safety.

Bob thought that in time his body would heal itself and he would be back to normal. Unfortunately, this was not the case. He experienced a continual sense of pain. He found himself unable to do the things he had taken for granted. He had difficulty playing with the kids, sleeping, or being sexual with his wife. A month after the accident, he paid a visit to his family physician, who could find no physical cause for his pain. The doctor gave him medication to help relieve the severe pain. For a while, the medication did the trick and it appeared that Bob was on the road to recovery. But eventually the pain got worse and he found that the medications didn't touch it.

Increasingly upset and fearful, he began taking days off from work. He became dependent on alcohol to help relieve his emotional and physical pain. His disposition gradually changed. He was easily upset by the presence of his own children, and his relationship with his wife deteriorated.

Eventually, Bob was dismissed from his job because he wasn't meeting company expectations. His drinking accelerated. He often exhibited bizarre behavior toward his children. They became afraid to be around their father. His relationship with his wife descended to physical abuse. Finally, she filed for divorce.

Before Bob was diagnosed as having chronic pain, he had already lost his family, job, and home. He had suffered severe psychological damage. This is an extreme example of the consequences of chronic pain but it is far from rare. Fortunately, most people seek help for their pain long before things unfold to that level.

One of the most difficult problems in dealing with chronic pain is that the physical sensation is not isolated to one specific place in the body. There is often a generalized feeling of pain that permeates the nerves, muscles or joints. The pain may sometimes become more intense in one part of the body one day and in another on the next. Beyond this, the emotions of anger, frustration and depression intensify pain so that it is difficult to isolate the level of pain or to reach an understanding of the difference between physical and emotional pain.

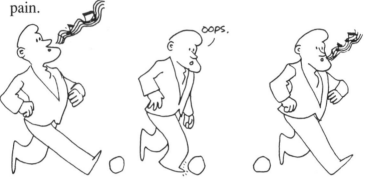

We have all had the experience of discovering a bruised toe without ever being aware of when it was bruised. Usually, this would have been a time when we were enthusiastically participating in an activity we enjoyed. At other times, of course, we are able to remember very clearly the pain and the event which caused it.

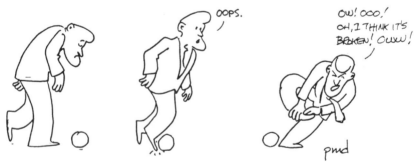

It is this unpredictability of where and when the pain will occur which is so difficult to understand. One factor which contributes to the unpredictable behavior of pain is the production of endorphins. Endorphins are chemicals secreted by the body which are natural pain killers. These often contribute to reduction of pain as well as to the sense of well-being which we experience after exercise, relaxation, or a particularly exciting activity.

But the production of these endorphins is not always predictable either. Since the conditions under which our bodies produce endorphins are tied to our mental state, there can be a wide variation in the amount of these amazing pain-killers which is produced at any given time. To help my clients experience this variation, I have them do a test. They pinch their wrist to cause a little discomfort. Then I take them through a series of basic breathing and relaxation exercises. At the end of the relaxation session, I have them pinch their wrist once again and ask them to compare the two sensations. If everyone responded alike, then everyone should notice a reduction in the pain at the second pinch.

Many say they experience less pain, others feel no change. Still others seem to experience greater pain. This variation demonstrates the fact that not everyone produces the same amount of endorphins under each circumstance. Those who had an abundant supply of endorphins experienced reduced pain. Those whose pain experience did not change, had not stimulated an endorphin release. The important point about this demonstration is that we begin to understand that not only is our pain is a very individual thing, but that it can be influenced not just by medications we swallow but by what we do with our bodies and our minds.

Beyond the complicated endorphin production process, however, there is something else which makes a difference. Our emotional state has a great effect on how we feel pain. For example, if we have undergone a major emotional trauma, our body retains that tension and stress. The result is that emotional trauma can intensify the experience of physical pain in such a way that our discomfort is increased well beyond what it would be if we were experiencing a serene and carefree existence. It makes sense, then, that if we can release the effects of that original emotional trauma, our pain levels will be reduced.

One client, for example, had multiple surgeries on his lower back. His pain extended well beyond the normal recovery time. As we began to work together, it became clear that there were blocks to his healing responses. As he followed the protocols which I use in working with chronic pain patients, he uncovered a deeply repressed anger over the severe physical abuse he had experienced from his father. During our healing sessions he was able to release that pent-up anger. His sensations of physical pain began to diminish when he understood that one source of the pain was the deep anger which had be suppressed for so long.

Among holistic practitioners, there is an increasing conviction that the cells in our body hold the energy pattern of the events that have taken place in our life. The belief is that as these patterns continue through the course of childhood, adolescence, and into adulthood, they become permanently stored in the body. At some point, the individual cannot contain such trauma and feelings and they begin to manifest themselves as physical symptoms.

When a crisis enters our life in the form of an accident, injury, or disease, the deep-rooted pain is unleashed and rises to the surface. The physical problem that evolves can be thought of as a symptom of the deeper emotional trauma. It is not enough, therefore, to treat only the physical symptoms. The stress of the emotional trauma remains and sends the pain signals to our brain even though the original emotional event has been forgotten or suppressed.

In order to find relief, then, we need to understand that pain is not simply a physical injury that can be healed or repaired. Understanding those fears which we often keep hidden even from ourselves is required.

Discovering these fears is not easy. Often, they have arisen from what we saw as a threat to our survival. For example, a child may see that a parent is angry and assume that the anger is a result of something the child has done. What may be happening is that the parent is angry over a quite unrelated matter but does not explain this to the child.

The child, meanwhile, is at a loss to know what behavior has created this anger and so feels only a vague and forboding guilt. This phenomena is not uncommon in divorces. A child may develop a sense of guilt over the failure of the parents' marriage although, in fact, the problems of the marriage were completely unrelated to the child. A child, however, lacks that perspective and the trauma of this guilt may lie buried deep in his or her psyche. As these emotional traumas accumulate, they can have serious consequences in later life.

Of the issues that tend to contribute to chronic pain in the clients I see, one of the most common is the perception of abuse in its many forms. The problem of abuse is that it always seems to be something that someone else does or that happens to someone else. We rarely apply it to our own experiences until we find ourselves in a position such that we can look at our lives from a new point of view. Then we begin to see that we may have experienced abuse and, just as important, that we may have been guilty of abusing others without realizing it. It is worthwhile, then, to take some time to outline some ways of looking at abuse.

An example of unintended abuse might be parents scolding children for never listening, never doing anything right, or always breaking things. Taken one at a time, these seem harmless enough. But they are messages. As these messages pile up, one negative accusation after another, a child begins to build a self-image of failure and unworthiness. The parent, throughout this time, has no intention of communicating such a message. The parent sees himself or herself as simply trying to correct unacceptable behavior. What is missing, of course, are the messages which applaud the child's achievements, the comment on the combed hair, the compliment on the room which is nicely cleaned up, the pleasure in a good grade at school. These are the positive messages which we need to balance those negative messages that we are all doomed to receive.

All of us have, at one time or another, experienced such unintended abuse. It is only when it becomes extreme and repetitive that it creates a problem for us. However, abuse can take on serious and devastating proportions when we are involved with persons who have serious problems of their own.

Such abuse falls into four general categories: Emotional Abuse, Physical Abuse, Sexual Abuse and Spiritual Abuse. These are frequent sources of chronic pain.

Emotional Abuse may take the form of the parental criticism described above which can have a serious impact on a child. But there are other harsher and more debilitating forms of abuse. A husband who continually criticizes his wife's performance in the kitchen, in bed, and to their friends, can reduce her self-esteem to serious levels of depression.

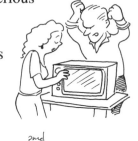

A woman who damages a man's sense of manhood by saying that he is not providing adequate support or comparing him unfavorably to her father or other males has the same effect. An older brother who robs his younger brother of his self-worth by calling him hurtful names increases the sense of unworthiness and contributes to a sense of depression.

Physical Abuse is about the inability to respond to physical violence. Like emotional abuse, it scars the individual pysche. The beating of an infant that has no way of responding to this trauma, the husband in an alcoholic rage who physically traumatizes his family, the frustrated mother who allows her anger to be expressed in uncontrolled beating of her child — all of these leave a deep and unexpressed anger in the unconscious.

Sexual Abuse is about a sexual act forced upon someone. It is often accompanied with physical and emotional violence leaving its victim helpless and unable to respond. This abuse can occur at any age. A man who has intercourse with his daughter telling her that he is teaching her to become a woman, a girl being raped on her way home from school, the older brother forcing a younger brother or sister into performing sexual acts are all experiences which leave anger, hurt, and a heavy overlay of guilt. These feelings are often hidden from the individual's conscious awareness.

Spiritual Abuse is about using religion for personal power rather than for the good of the people. An extreme example would be the tragedy of the Jonestown Massacre where over seven hundred people, following the orders of their leader, drank a poisoned drink. The tragedy of the David Koresh sect in Waco, Texas where men, women, and children died in a stand-off with governmental authorities is another sad incident. Church members who are manipulated by church officials for personal gain suffer from spiritual abuse when they discover that the person they admired and trusted has betrayed them in the name of a spiritual cause.

Abuse can have fearful consequences on our physical health but there is another issue that can leave the body at risk of chronic pain. That issue is the fear of abandonment. As infants and young children, we are totally dependent on others to take care of us. A thread of fear runs through all of us that those who we depend on for survival needs will desert us. We all feel a pressure to please others so that they will not leave us. Gradually, as our own self-confidence grows, this pressure is reduced but we are never totally free of the the fear of abandonment. The consequence is that when we experience the separation from someone who is important to us, the potential for trauma exists. The loss of a parent through death, divorce, or desertion often leaves children fearful and insecure. They search within themselves for the reason why they were left alone. Often this results in a deep-seated and unexpressed feeling of unworthiness. These traumatic experiences, too, are stored in the memory of the cell and may emerge later in an apparently unrelated physical problem.

All these experiences result in our fear, and ultimately, our anger at having our life expectations violated. Because on the surface, this anger seems irrational, it is often submerged and held in the body. Much later, it emerges to block the energy that allows the body to heal.

What then is the task that faces those of us who experience chronic pain? We must be open to the possibility that some suppressed anger, fear, or guilt, may exist in our body as stress. We must allow ourselves to explore the idea that an underlying trauma lies at the root of our physical pain. As we search for such incidents, there are many therapists who can help us. The choice of therapist is an intensely individual one and will be discussed later. It is enough to note here that we need not do all this work without help. But whether we perform our own self-analysis or find others to help us, it is important to confront those long hidden and suppressed feelings because they are preventing us from healing as we should. Some of us will never accept that there is an emotional component of our pain. If that is the case, we will spend our time searching for medications and medical discoveries to reduce our discomfort.

Those of us who are open to new options will search within ourselves for an understanding of these emotional blocks to our healing. As we become aware of these emotions, the physical pain may diminish, and we will begin to view our pain from a new perspective.

Questions for Consideration:

◆ *Is part of my frustration over my pain, that I am not distinguising between acute and chronic pain?*

◆ *When I think of how and when my pain began, can I pinpoint any emotional crisis or stress points that may have complicated my healing?*

◆ *How do I feel about the idea that my pain may have an emotional base? Am I ready to explore that possibility?*

◆ *Are there abuse or abandonment issues in my life that may be a source of suppressed anger or fear?*

- 3 -

Pain and Our Emotions

The relationship of pain to emotional trauma is at the core of this approach to healing. As we have seen, emotional trauma can be as dramatic as rape, or as subtle as emotional abandonment. Any of these traumas affect the way we feel pain as it develops in the body. When the person who has repressed a deep emotional trauma experiences physical pain, the intensity of that pain matches the intensity of the repressed emotion. As we find ways to uncover this hidden trauma, we may be surprised to find that our pain could increase. But as the process unfolds, and we deal with those emotions which have been so long suppressed, physical pain subsides.

In this complicated process, we often are unable to distinguish that part of the pain which is physical from that which is emotional. As the pinch test illustrated, emotional states have an effect on the endorphins which affect how we experience pain. It is important, therefore, to work on both emotional as well as physical symptoms even though we cannot always separate the two. By this I mean that when we find we are in a state of high stress, our experience of pain becomes more intense as well. We can reduce that level of stress through relaxation and breathing exercises and find some relief even as we find antidotes for our physical pain. As we begin to release deep-seated emotional trauma, additional relief can develop without our ever being able to identify specifically, which treatment was most effective. We will simply find that both emotional and physical relief evolve as we continue our healing pilgrimage. The following case will illustrate how this works.

Lisa came to my office, unable to understand why she had such terrible pain. In spite of multiple surgeries, the pain persisted. She had attended other pain programs and had been heavily medicated with pain-relievers and anti-depressants. As we began a discussion of her life, she remembered that her father had suffered with chronic pain as well.

Her father could not express emotional feelings because he believed them to be inappropriate. His physical pain became the symptom of these emotions. As we talked, she realized that without being aware of it, she had included in her own life, her father's beliefs. She had ignored and suppressed her anger and hurt feelings because she had learned from her father that such emotions were not appropriate. For a very long time, she had presented a facade of contentment to her husband, children, and friends. She discounted her feelings and deeper needs and focused on the needs of others.

A series of accidents throughout her life had resulted in a painful spinal condition. In addition, her carpal tunnel syndrome was threatening to make continued work impossible. The repression of emotions was having the same effect in her life as it had her father's.

Like her father, Lisa had always feared that if she expressed her feelings, she would be abandoned. But by not expressing her feelings, they remained with her and filled her with anger at her parents, siblings and friends because they had failed to sense the hurts and fears she was suffering.

Lisa had had to care for her bed-ridden father for some time. At the time, she felt that she was only doing what was expected of her and that she should be pleased that she could help. As time went on, however, she found herself needing to suppress an anger over how she was trapped in this situation. On the one hand, she felt the anger at how this limited her own life and on the other she felt guilt at what she believed was an unacceptable selfishness. As all this was taking place, her back pain had intensified. Only now, in therapy, was she able to see the connection between her back pain and the suppressed anger.

Once Lisa began to deal with these feelings, her emotional turmoil increased but her physical pain diminished. As her therapy continued, she began to accept the new insights that she had uncovered and, with this acceptance, her emotional pain also subsided. Life no longer seemed a dead end of pain and frustration. She began to feel confident about dealing with her life situations.

Pain caused by hidden emotional trauma can be tricky. It can wear all types of masks and take on all sorts of disguises. It may hide in lost memories, or in situations that are too painful to remember. Often they are tucked away and stored neatly out of one's conscious awareness. These memories are difficult to recognize, let alone to acknowledge.

Steve's experience is an example of deeply stored painful memories. At the time of his accident, Steve was living in the fast lane. He was a workaholic, holding down two jobs so he could afford the better things in life. He was able to pay his mortgage and make the payments on his car and boat. He arranged to put money away for retirement, vacations, and his children's college education. He tried to give his children the things that he himself felt deprived of. This life-style appeared to work well for Steve until he injured himself at his drill press. His injury was serious enough that he was prevented from continuing his work on his second job. Confronted with intense physical pain and the growing fear of financial ruin, he desperately searched in the medical community for an answer to his problem.

Steve, for whom work was the center of life, was faced with the fact that he could no longer perform the job which was so important to him. The resulting depression drove him to therapy. Unaware of the inner turmoil which possessed him, he had locked away the memory of the physical beatings and emotional upheavals which had shaped his view of himself. During his therapy, he took the time to allow these memories to surface. He recognized that the emphasis on work and accumulating material things was an attempt to go beyond the sense of unworthiness which he had learned from the childhood abuse. He confronted, for the first time as an adult, those feelings of unworthiness and he saw them quite differently now. He realized that he had accepted someone else's view of his value and had never questioned it. As a result, he was driven to prove that he was worthy. He found that as he worked on a more positive view of himself the emotional stress as well as the physical pain began to fade.

Lisa and Steve are good examples of how emotional trauma can be hidden. This stress that they learned to hold in so well took on the physical form of mishaps, accidents, and painful relationships. Because this process is so complicated, it may be helpful to develop a way of thinking about how emotional trauma has a physical effect on our bodies. This understanding can be helpful in visualizing the process at work in our own bodies.

Emotions and the Distortion of the Life Force

To begin with, we must think of the body as something more than muscle, bone, and tissue. As anyone who has ever seen a raw beef roast knows, something has changed between the time that beef roast was part of a powerful steer running in the field and the limp cold bit of flesh on the kitchen table. That difference can be described in many ways but the phrases, "life force" and "life energy" seem to describe best what has been lost. Regardless of what our religious beliefs are, we intuitively know that there is an energy running through living things. If we say that this life energy animates or gives life to our collection of cells, bones, and blood, it follows that when this "energy" flows freely through the body, we are in good health. But when something blocks this energy, the body is susceptible to illness, disease, and injury.

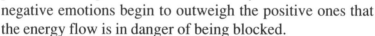

Emotions can influence the flow of this energy. Anger, stress, and fear impede the flow; happiness, love, and contentment enhance it. Ordinarily, the body can adjust to the flow of positive and negative emotions. It is only when negative emotions begin to outweigh the positive ones that the energy flow is in danger of being blocked.

Early in our childhood we begin to collect experiences of fear, pain, and danger. Usually, we express these experiences in the security of our parent's love and care. However, if we are not able to express our fears or pain and we do not receive the comfort which releases them, the memory of the fear lies buried in our mind and body. If there are many of these, the hidden stress begins to make us vulnerable to physical symptoms in the form of illness or pain. As children, safety is our highest priority. Any time we believe that our environment is not safe, we try to protect ourselves. The stress of an angry parent, the fear of abandonment, or the experience of physical pain may create desperate emotions which are not dispelled when the immediate problem is over. We may come to believe that the anger of our parents is a normal state that somehow we have caused. And if that anger occurs once, it can occur again. We become confused about our parent's actions. We find that the same hand that loves, nurtures, and caresses us can become a violent weapon of pain, misery, and punishment.

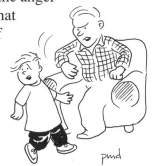

pmd

We store these emotions within the cells of our body and they remain there as a potential physical problem. We learn quickly that to show certain emotions, sexual expressions, and feelings is prohibited. But we do not learn how to release these emotions in an acceptable way.

As the body and mind learn to store these feelings in various locations, our free flow of life energy is restricted. When this pattern continues through the course of our childhood, adolescence, and into adulthood, these patterns become habitual. One day we can no longer contain the trauma and it begins to manifest itself in physical symptoms. These symptoms can take the form of an accident, injury, or disease. When that happens, we confront these emotions for the first time in many years. We can either suppress them again, or take an opportunity to explore and, finally, release them. Exploring these underlying emotions can be the beginning of healing.

So there are two levels at which emotions have an effect on our experience of pain. The first and most superficial is the way emotions and stress can intensify our experience of pain, regardless of whether it is acute or chronic pain. We can diminish the intensity of the pain by using relaxation techniques to reduce the emotional and physical stress of our body.

The second level is the suppressed emotions or memories of trauma that operate below our conscious level. These are the emotions which remain hidden until the body experiences a physical or emotional trauma that triggers the alarm system of pain that continues to sound long after the physical problem has been solved. This is the chronic pain that continues in maddeningly unexplainable ways. If this is the source of the pain, we must not expect relief from medical treatment alone. We must begin to look for the underlying emotional trauma that is creating the pain.

The healing process, then, begins with a new way of thinking about ourselves. We should try to see ourselves not as a patients delivering our bodies to the medical profession but as healers who are able to make a difference in our own state of health. This does not mean that we are alone in this effort. It means that we begin with our own sense of ourselves and our past, and we reach out to the health-care world for help in our healing. We must think of our healing path as a search for coaches who can help us with one or another of our concerns in the way a professional athlete looks for coaches to improve one aspect of his game. He may have many coaches for many different problems, but he has one goal in mind. He wants to improve his whole game. In the same way, our goal is a healthy life which is not encumbered by pain. In this search, we do not expect the goal to be reached through the help of one coach only, we accept what is helpful and move on. We begin by defining our needs through self analysis. We continue to evaluate our progress and find coaches to help us with new aspects of our problems until we reach our goal of a healthy life. We have followed the path of *healing* not *curing*.

Questions for Consideration:

♦ *When I think of the moments in my life when I was overcome with fear, hurt or anger, is there a connection between that time and the beginnings of my chronic pain?*

♦ *Is there some place in my body which seems to store that fear, hurt or anger?*

- 4 -

Victims of Pain

We have seen how the brain receives the warning signals from the nerve endings in the body and we have discussed how emotional stress can increase the feeling of that pain when it is experienced. In the last chapter we discussed how the body stores memories of emotional trauma below our conscious awareness, only to have it burst out when there is an onset of another traumatic experience.

The question is, why don't we just remember the pain and release it? Why don't we express our emotional feelings and let them go? Why do we hold it all in until it breaks out of its own accord? Psychologists have pondered that question for many years and they have arrived at many different explanations. The general answer is that we play many roles in society. We learn that certain behavior is appropriate for certain people in different circumstances. In this society, for example, we learn that if we are males we should not cry or show emotion unless it is anger in preparation for a battle. If we are females, we learn that we should not be too aggressive. We should try to get what we want by pleasing others. Neither one of these attitudes is likely to help us express our hurt feelings or fear. So we find ways to hide it, often from ourselves as well. We should consider beliefs such as these which we have held, unquestioningly, and ask ourselves whether the belief makes sense for us now and whether it has the potential to block our healing energy.

Very early, we try to get feedback from the world around us about "who we really are." As we grow in that understanding, we also recognize that we can give feedback to others about "who *they* really are." As these personal relationships grow, they take on certain characteristics. One person seems to dominate the other. For example, a parent exercises great control over a small child, not only from the standpoint of size, but also because the parent controls the necessities of life available to that child. But these roles are not set in stone. They begin to change as the child grows older. Adolescence is the period in which children begin to experiment with how they can control their own lives as well as the lives of others.

This brief outline is meant only to suggest the way in which we learn and grow and adapt to the circumstances that shape our attitudes about ourselves. As we develop we begin to accept certain ideas about who we are. These ideas become our reality. This is the point at which we begin to accept limitations on ourselves. We decide we cannot be terrific basketball players. We cannot be beauty queens. We will never be good students. We will never be good with mechanical things. But at the same time we are learning what we can be. We can be good pianists, good sons or daughters whose mother loves us, brothers or sisters who help the whole family. We can be a good cooks, or terrific comics at parties. We receive messages from others, accept the ideas without question, and do what we can to fulfill the expectations. It is through this process that we can become victims as well as victimizers.

All of us make sacrifices for others out of love, respect, and sometimes fear. However, when we allow these sacrifices to take over our lives, we lose our individuality. We accept the role of the sacrificer to the exclusion of all other roles. We come to believe that our worthiness is dependent on the sacrifices we make for others. When this happens, we have allowed ourselves to become victims.

It is important to understand why we might become victims. Often we see this as our only option for survival. Our experiences often lead us to believe that we are made worthy only through the praise of others. When this praise is not forthcoming, we have no sense of self-worth. When we face criticism, we feel diminished in painful ways. These experiences make us dependent on others for our own identity. We make ourselves victims of those people whose praise we seek. The following example will illustrate this process.

Margery came to me in severe pain as a result of fibromy-algia. Our introductory discussion revealed that she felt that she had no way to change her life circumstances. Her husband seemed to believe that her pain was an excuse for not meeting his expectations. Her children, absorbed in their own lives, left her with a feeling that she was all alone. She lived for a word of praise from her husband which never came. Nevertheless, she continued to do things to please him, sacrificing her own needs.

As she explored her situation in therapy, she discovered that she had unconsciously chosen this victim state because it was only as a victim that she was able to feel worthy. As this understanding grew, she tried to increase her sense of worthiness through ways which were not dependent on the opinions of others. She found that she had many abilities that were valuable in themselves, but which she had dismissed because others appeared not to value them. Gradually she found that she was able to assert herself in her relationship with her husband. Together they were able to work out a healthier relationship and her deep seated anger was released. She replaced the anger with the ability to direct her emotions to healthier outlets and the physical pain began to subside.

On the surface, it seems unreasonable that we would willingly submit ourself to being victims. We cannot ignore, however, the power of deep, fundamental needs, in the human psyche. As infants, we respond to love, care, and approval. And if any of these are withheld, we will do whatever is necessary to fill the void. Sometimes what we do appears unreasonable to others, but if it works, we do it. My own experience illustrates this behavior.

As a child I had difficulty in maintaining a sense of self-worth. It seemed to me that I never measured up. When I received only average grades in school, I felt that I had not met the family's expectations. The effect of any disciplinary measures I received was to confirm that I was inadequate. The one activity to which I gave my all was ice hockey. But even though I considered myself competitive with other players, I did not feel that I received the acknowledgment that would have confirmed my sense of self-worth.

One day while I was playing hockey, I got hit with a puck just above the eye. The resulting wound required five stitches. Because of the shock, I felt no pain. However, I was dumfounded by the attention I received from the members of my team, my coach, my family, and my friends. They treated me as if I were a hero. In this experience, I had found a surrogate for self-worth.

For the first time I found that pain was a valuable commodity. I am not sure that I consciously worked out this plan, but the experience reinforced the positive benefits of pain. As I look back on many years of emotional and physical difficulties, I now realize that I have used pain as a method of survival.

To survive, we all need a sense of self-worth and, if necessary, we find it outside ourselves. I see now that I became a martyr to emotional distress and physical pain inflicted by others because in the martyrdom, I found a substitute for self-worth. What I did not understand was that I was victimizing myself.

We are potential victims when we become desperate to find something which will make us feel better about ourselves. In this struggle, we become vulnerable to manipulation by others. We are continually searching for something to do for others so that we will receive the praise and recognition which does not seem to come from other parts of our lives. We are vulnerable because others can withold that all-important praise and leave the victim devastated.

What is puzzling is the fact that as victims, we are not completely conscious of our actions. We become programmed to behave in the role of the victim. We are manipulated and we manipulate. We sacrifice ourselves to appease others. We believe we have no choice.

It is not uncommon to exhibit victim behavior in one form or another. The very core of this victimization begins in our own thought process long before anything happens outside in the physical world.

My view of my own inadequacies led to my using injuries in sports to find gratification. My reward was a little more attention from others. I found myself in situations in which I was rendered powerless in my personal relationships with my family, friends and business associates. As a child and as an adult, I would find myself playing the role of the scapegoat.

By becoming the victim, no matter what the outcome, I didn't have to be responsible for my actions. I discovered that although I was powerless, I could use victimization to my advantage by manipulating others to get what I wanted. By becoming a victim, I derived great benefits for my own personal survival and satisfaction. However the law of cause and effect eventually caught up with me.

As my personal and business life deteriorated, I was forced to face the fact that only I could create a true sense of self-worth. Fortunately, I found a way to do that. When I learned to face the problems which confronted me and accept my part in creating them, I was able gain the necessary distance to separate myself from my victimhood.

In my practice, I have discovered that I was not alone in this scenario. Many of my clients have come to me with similar stories. Those who discover the nature of their own victimization are firmly set on the road to their own recovery.

Cheryl, for example, came for treatment for back pain resulting from an automobile accident. The doctors could not explain why the pain persisted. During therapy she experienced a flashback of sexual abuse at an early age by her father. As she confronted the issue of the abuse and how it influenced her later experiences, she began to see the connection with her use of drugs, her suicide attempts, her failed relationships, and her lack of self-worth. Once she began to understand that her pain was a symptom of that early victimization, she was able to develop a healthy sense of self-worth through the release of pent-up emotion. As this emotional trauma was released, the chronic pain diminished.

The more I work with chronic pain clients, the more I see clusters of belief systems that work against the healing process. These belief systems are not something that we arrive at consciously. They depend much more on our experiences as children and adolescents. Sometimes they are habits of thought which we adopted in a moment of crisis but have stayed with us long after the crisis has passed. They are characterized by the attitude of the victim, and they arise from a sense of being powerless to achieve what we need.

As I review the cases of my clients as well as my own life, I can see the difference between people who somehow develop belief systems which lead them into a victim role and other people who have avoided these beliefs. It is clear to me that these victim beliefs have delayed my healing process. I include them here so that others may examine their own lives for these clusters of beliefs prevent progress in healing.

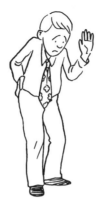

Victim Beliefs

◆ *Work is the only means I have to earn the appreciation and respect of others which is so important to me.*

◆ *Giving to others will make me valuable to them.*

◆ *Being a martyr keeps me safe.*

◆ *My friends prove that they are really my friends when they appreciate my pain.*

◆ *I am important to my family only because of what I do for them.*

◆ *People can be manipulated to get me what I need.*

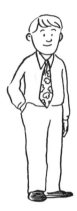

Non-Victim Beliefs

◆ *Work in and of itself is self-fulfilling.*

◆ *In valuing myself I can help others.*

◆ *I am secure because I understand my own strengths.*

◆ *My friendships are enhanced by a mutual recognition of the value of each other's qualities.*

◆ *My family's love is a given. It need not be earned.*

◆ *I have the ability to meet my own needs.*

As we perform our self-analysis regarding these beliefs, it is important to remember that the victim state is an extreme point on a continuum of normal behavior. We all make sacrifices for others, and we are right to feel better about ourselves because of that.

The difference between Victims and Non-Victims is that the sense of self-worth for Non-Victims arises from a confident belief in their own abilities and value. Unlike Victims, their opinion of themselves is not dependent on the sacrifices they make. Victims, on the other hand, cling to the belief that they are worthy *only* through self-sacrifice.

Questions for Consideration:

♦ *When I think about my identity, what qualities do I have that I value? Who led me to value those qualities?*

♦ *What are the qualities or abilities I lack? What experiences or people led me to believe I don't have them and I can't attain them?*

♦ *When I look back from this distance, are those people right?*

♦ *Do I have victim beliefs which are limiting me?*

- 5 -

The Chronic Pain Profiles

There is another part of our behavior which has a bearing on how we allow ourselves to heal. That is the way we try to defend ourselves from those unpleasant or painful experiences which beset us all. Whether this pain arises from abandonment, powerlessness, or simply a low self-image, we find ways to protect ourselves from it. If we have been badly hurt by unkind words, we can protect ourselves by attacking others before they attack us. If we have been convinced that we can do nothing for ourselves, it is likely that we will demand that others help us without even attempting the task. For those of us with chronic pain, abandonment issues are very common. The feeling of being abandoned is one of the most fearful experiences we have. Abandonment means that the support we depended on has disappeared. As small children, if our parent or care-giver disappeared without some explanation of when they would return, we reacted with instant fear. As we grow older, most of us form a world in which we try to insure that the support we think we need will be there. When we are abandoned, we are frightened by this new world in which the support we had always expected has disappeared. This sense of isolation is difficult to face, and we all confront the need to protect ourselves from this painful and frightening experience.

This protection may take different forms in different personalities but they all have the common purpose of repressing the emotional trauma that underlies our pain. People appear to follow several patterns of behavior in developing their defense against these traumatic emotions. While we all adopt some defensive roles to insulate us from emotional trauma, when these defenses become a deeply imbedded pattern of behavior, a danger develops that the defense will prevent a healthy flow of healing energy and the exploration of new possibilities.

A study of these defense patterns reveals a set of profiles which characterize the way we defend ourselves from our emotional trauma. The profiles presented here are based on an analysis formulated by Alexander Lowen, John Pierrakos, and Barbara Ann Brennan. The descriptive categories have been reshaped to apply specifically to people with chronic pain.

As we review these profiles, we must remember that these individual characteristics are present in all of us to some degree. However, if the cluster of characteristics appears to be the only means we use to cope with our issues, such a profile could inhibit the healing process. These profiles are offered here, not as labels for behavior or beliefs that we cannot change, but rather as a way to look at one part of our personality that may become a hindrance rather than a help. When we recognize ourselves in these descriptions, we need to ask ourselves where that belief system came from and what other choices do we have. When we recognize that one type of defense is being carried to an extreme in our lives, we can use these descriptions to understand and change that behavior or the belief on which the behavior is based.

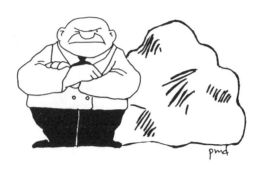

The Rock

The Rock has the virtue of being solid and unchanging. But sometimes, this becomes a problem rather than a virtue. When we turn ourselves into rocks, we create the following limitations in healing ourselves:

◆ *"Rocks" only accept traditional methods.*

◆ *"Rocks" are not open to other possible treatments.*

◆ *"Rocks" limit themselves to the recommendation of only one authority.*

◆ *"Rocks" avoid connecting emotional trauma to pain.*

◆ *"Rocks" are quick to dismiss treatments which do not have immediate results.*

◆ *"Rocks" blame others for their pain.*

◆ *"Rocks" tend to be resistant to treatments which are new or different or which create unfamiliar emotions or experiences.*

In our first meeting, Linda demonstrated many of these "rock" characteristics. As she listened to my description of possible therapies, she seemed uncomfortable making the choice for herself. She had always expected specialists to make these decisions for her. Although she continued therapy for a while, she never really accepted the idea that there might be an emotional component in her pain because she had always thought of pain as being only physical. Even as the therapy began to uncover emotional trauma, she failed to connect it to her pain. In fact, she decided that the emotional discomfort proved that the therapy was not effective, so she terminated the therapy after a short time.

Months later, she returned. Her pain had become so severe that, in desperation, she tried some of the recommended exercises. Because she experienced positive results, she returned to the therapy with a new attitude. Linda was finally able to find a way to break through the resistance and release her emotional trauma.

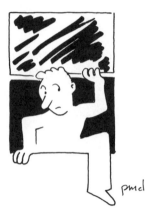

The Escape Artist:

Escape Artists have the quality of quicksilver. They can move instantly to many different realities. This provides them with a wide range of experiences and insights. But they often find themselves unable to confront the serious problems which must be resolved. Their fear drives them to escape through the following types of behavior:

- ◆ *"The Escape Artist" uses fantasy to avoid confrontations.*

- ◆ *"The Escape Artist" focuses on what the future might have been and what has been lost thus avoiding the present moment.*

- ◆ *"The Escape Artist" focuses on what the future could be if there were no pain.*

♦ *"The Escape Artist" forms elaborate plans to avoid uncomfortable physical and emotional situations.*

Peter, a classic "Escape Artist" suffering from lower back pain, had great difficulty in focusing on his present pain. He spent a lot of time talking about what his life had been like before the accident. He complained about lost opportunities in his business and relationships. He postponed suggested healing strategies saying that he would try them when he felt better. As treatment continued and emotional issues arose, he avoided experiencing the emotions by intellectually analyzing them rather than allowing the feelings to emerge and be experienced directly.

It was some time before he realized that his avoidance behavior was obstructing his healing. Only when he learned to concentrate on the present moment and experience it at an emotional level, was he able to make progress in his healing.

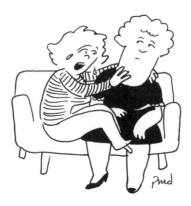

The Clinging Vine:

For most of us, accepting the help of others makes us uncomfortable. Too often, we feel we have to do it all ourselves. In many cases, if we were to allow others to help us, we would be better off. But there is a point when accepting help from others becomes a problem. This usually occurs when our own self-concept has deteriorated to the point that we feel powerless to help ourselves. We desperately cling to others to survive. This dependence can have serious consequences for the healing process. The following behavior marks the profile of a "Clinging Vine".

◆ *"The Clinging Vine" uses pain as a means of connecting to others.*

◆ *"The Clinging Vine" uses pain as a means of self-identity.*

♦ *"The Clinging Vine" defines pain in negative terms.*

♦ *"The Clinging Vine" often provokes irritation in others as a desperate way of attracting attention.*

Jill was a classic Clinging Vine. In addition to injuries resulting from a car accident, she experienced both work-related and domestic abuse. No matter how hard she tried, she continually found herself in uncomfortable situations. The only positive social relationships she maintained were with the health care professionals whom she saw weekly. She desperately searched among friends and medical professionals for the sympathy which would affirm her self-worth. She was cooperative and interested in her therapy, but when she left the treatment center, she returned to a world which did not provide the support she depended on. She became a frequent complainer and alienated many of her acquaintances by implying that they had failed her. Because of her dependence on the attitudes of others, her healing progress was delayed. As her therapy continued, we worked to make her feel less dependent. Gradually, she began to see that she could control her own destiny. She is now seeking help in getting out of her abusive environment which was not conducive to her healing process.

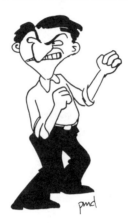

The Shark:

The active and aggressive approach to problem solving that often seems necessary in the business world today can have a down-side when it is applied to personal life situations. The behavior of "The Shark" in seeking healing is often self-defeating.

- ◆ *"The Shark" blames others for lack of relief and for not being sympathetic.*

- ◆ *"The Shark" doesn't trust others.*

- ◆ *"The Shark" views the system as predatory.*

- ◆ *"The Shark" builds a defense of anger.*

- ◆ *"The Shark" likes to be in charge and is suspicious of cooperative activities.*

♦ *"The Shark" finds reasons for not pursuing self-recovery.*

♦ *"The Shark" asserts power to preserve a sense of individuality.*

Frank lost no time in demonstrating his "Shark" behavior when he arrived in the program. He was angry at his doctors whom he believed had failed to provide the appropriate therapy. He was angry at the amount of paper work required by the insurance company. And he was angry at his boss for not holding his job. He viewed our therapies with suspicion. Rather than participate in the exercises, he demanded pain medications. When these were denied, he systematically alienated the staff by implying that they were preventing him from getting pain relief.

As the program continued, Frank found a therapist who was able to help him confront the reality of his situation. Once he saw that his therapy depended on his own actions and that the staff was open to discussing his concerns, he was willing to participate in the healing program. Anger as a defense was no longer necessary.

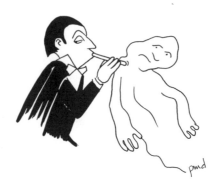

The Vampire

The flattering interest which "The Vampire" first demonstrates in forming a relationship, begins to be suffocating and draining, as it becomes clear that this is not a relationship in which energy is exchanged. "The Vampire" has no energy to spare and must depend on the energy of others:

◆ *"The Vampire" uses the energy of others for comfort.*

◆ *"The Vampire" is a doctor-shopper taking whatever energy is allowed and moving on.*

◆ *"The Vampire" finds short-term relief through therapy but does not expect it to last.*

◆ *"The Vampire" always feels that there is never enough of anything.*

George was a business executive. He was a typical "type A" personality. His chronic pain had persisted through numerous operations, and he did not hesitate to explain that the many doctors with whom he consulted could not diagnose his situation. The characteristic "Vampire" behavior became evident as he explained that he was a victim of fate. He did not connect his deep depressions to his chronic pain or his continued ill health. He searched out treatments in which he expected and received short-term relief but when emotional issues began to emerge, he moved on to another treatment.

In his self-analysis during the therapy, George was confronted with this issue. Gradually, he came to understand that he had a part in his own healing, and that the energy of others would not bring about permanent recovery. As he began to examine the underlying issues that drove his anger, his healing began. Ultimately he was able to confront and experience his emotions which opened up a new healing possibilities.

In reviewing these personality profiles, we can all find in them behavior that we recognize as our own. This does not mean that we need to accept that label ourselves. It does mean that we must recognize those behaviors which are preventing us from exploring new healing techniques.

Questions for Consideration:

◆ *As I read these profiles, did I recognize examples of any of them among people I know?*

◆ *Can I see ways in which those people are limited by their personality profile?*

◆ *Do I have some of the characteristics of one or more of these profile types?*

◆ *If so, am I limiting my possibilities in healing because of my approach to life?*

◆ *Is there something I can do about it?*

◆ *Are there characteristics in these lists that particularly disturb me? If so, why?*

- 6 -

Taking Command of Our Healing

The previous chapters have provided background and ideas about the nature of the healing process. They are not intended to provide hard and fast rules to a guaranteed recovery. Rather, they are intended to stimulate ideas to which each person will respond in his or her own way. A major theme in this book is that we carry within ourselves the ability to recognize our own healing path. I do not mean that we ignore the advice of the medical community. In most cases, that advice makes excellent sense. But we must insist that we understand what the treatment is intended to do and, when we are offered choice of treatments, we listen to the ideas of the medical professional and make our decision based on our own intuitive sense of what is right for us.

This may be an unfamiliar approach to those who have grown used to a health care system which diagnoses, recommends therapies, and accepts and rejects clients based on a pre-established criteria. While that system is effective in short-term injury and illness, it is less effective when the illness has been complicated by emotional trauma.

For those of us with chronic pain, that is very often the case. Many times, we have exhausted the traditional therapies without finding relief. It is only when we can take command of our healing that we can devise the necessary healing process.

Intuition is a key component in taking command of our healing. I am not speaking here of a minor whim but rather a recognition or a deep sense of "knowing" that a certain strategy or technique is appropriate for us. We have all experienced this "knowing," but we are most aware of it when we have ignored it. Who has not exclaimed at one time or another, *I knew I should have done that!* But the realization that our intuition was right comes only when we have made the wrong choice.

For most of us, learning to listen to our intuition is not an easy task. We have been taught most of our life that we need to make decisions based on "facts." We need to develop a clear, rational argument to support our decisions. I do not disagree with this when the "facts" are clear, and the arguments can be presented without bias or fear. But in everyday life, the number of decisions in which this is possible is minimal. "Facts" turn out to be "appearances." Arguments are weighted with the self-interest of one or more of our competing desires. The selection of one choice really may be based on our need to please our family and friends rather than what we really believe. For example, we may have a relative who has a medical background and she insists that we should consult a specific specialist. Our intuition may suggest another approach but because our relative has the force of authority, we agree to that choice. Or the choice may be made because it makes the most financial sense. For example, we follow a certain therapy even though it appears not to be beneficial but it is the only treatment our insurance will pay for.

Such reasoning is not appropriate when the decision involves a concern for our own health. When our health is at stake, we really must take more personal stock of the situation. Our first step in doing this is to begin to know ourselves and to recognize that voice within us which speaks with confidence about our best interests.

To have confidence in that voice, we first must recognize the other voices which are providing competing advice. These voices are the learned voices of fear, of a low self-image, of a need to please others, or defenses like "The Rock," "The Clinging Vine," and all the others we discussed in the last chapter. We must learn to still those voices and listen, then, to the remaining inner knowledge which we all possess.

It is not the intention of this book to prescribe a single way of doing this. Some people do this easily. They seem, automatically, to act on their "hunches," to know what they want to do and when they want to do it. Others have been trained to ignore their own hunches and search, instead, for "authorities" who can tell them what to do. Others have given up and simply follow whatever advice is offered, regardless of its source.

To retrieve this intuition, we first must begin to value ourselves and recognize that self-interest is not the same as selfishness. We then must ask ourselves, quietly and alone, to hear the inner voice. If we are having problems with stilling those competing voices, we must confront them with our own self-analysis. We must look at our belief about ourselves and question how we have arrived at those beliefs. If the answers to those questions lead us to a different view of ourselves, we must have the courage to accept it.

Next we must review our beliefs about our illness or pain. We must explain to ourselves how this illness or pain arose in our lives. What emotional circumstances surrounded that event? What is the illness or pain preventing us from doing? Is this illness or pain, in some way, shielding us from some unpleasant circumstance that we would have to face if we were not ill?

Finally, having confronted ourselves and our illness and pain, we must now look clearly at our choices for healing. What has to be changed if we are to heal? What medical options are available? How will they help us? What emotional traumas need to be confronted and released? How will we do these things?

These questions and answers are personal and private. We, ourselves, decide whether we will discuss them with others. Some people find the simple act of explaining their decisions to another person gives that decision power. Others prefer to make their decisions in private and present only the confidence in their decisions to others. The program described in Part Two suggests that we keep a journal so that we can track our own development. As we grow in our self-analysis, and as we experience the various healing techniques, the journal will provide us with a companion for our journey. We will have other companions as well. There will be the friends we wish to confide in. There will be the care givers and therapists with whom we can discuss parts of our healing journey, but our journal will reflect the entire path.

The purpose of Part One of this book is to suggest a way of thinking about chronic pain that takes into consideration all aspects of the experience. We have seen that our experience of pain, in the narrowest physical sense, is nothing more than an alarm system. We have seen that this alarm system can be shut off by anesthetic, by surgery and by stimulating endorphins through relaxation techniques. But we have also seen that our experience of pain is more than a pain impulse to the brain.

The pain impulse may be triggered not only by a damaged muscle, cell, or bone, but by the stress of everyday events. And beyond the "stress headache," for which we have an immediate explanation, there are the "memories" in the cells of emotional trauma which we have long since suppressed but which are now breaking out to demand relief.

Those of us with chronic pain must look to that latter explanation carefully. If the medical treatments which have already been tried have failed to shut off the alarm system, there is something more to be considered. We have a choice, here, as to whether to proceed or not.

We can insist that there is only a physical base for this pain and look for the most effective anesthetic we can find that will allow us to continue our lives, or we can explore the possibilities that alternative treatments can offer.

In either case, if we are making the decision with a clear understanding of the alternatives which are available to us, we are, indeed, *taking command of our healing*. It is only when we refuse to explore the possibilities that we resign that command to others.

Questions for Consideration:

◆ *Are there times in my life that I use my intuition successfully?*

◆ *What do I need to do to cultivate that ability?*

◆ *Am I ready to start this healing path?*

◆ *If not, what more do I need to do?*

Part Two:

Steps for Your

Healing Path...

- **Self Analysis**

- **Healing Exercises**

- **Transition to Health**

- 7 -

Self-Analysis

This section of the book presents a way to develop a plan for our own healing path. We will begin with the self-analysis we have been discussing. When we have identified our problems, we will be able to define the goals for our healing. With this understanding, we move on to exercises which will help us grow in our healing path. Beyond this, is a list of possible therapies from which to select our team of healing assistants. All of these suggestions remain simply that. We select only those ideas which seem to be appropriate in our healing program. The only essential part of the program is that we end with a plan that we have designed for our healing.

A Journal for the Journey To Healing

Since this is an exploration, we cannot always predict with certainty the path which we will take. Many people find keeping a journal helps them focus on their search. The questions on the following pages cover a broad range of concerns to be considered as we go. We can select these ideas or develop our own. Those people who find journal-writing unrewarding, may still benefit by allowing the ideas to play out in their mind before moving on to the next chapters.

Journal-writing is most effective when we schedule a specific time in the day to write in the journal. This has two benefits. First, we will be less likely to forget or skip the journal-writing if there is a time we habitually do the work. Secondly, both our conscious and our subconscious mind begin to store up ideas for the journal writing. This is not a conscious act, but when we begin writing, the ideas are there!

Every journal has an audience. The audience for this journal is ourselves. We are not writing for anyone else nor do we intend to show the journal to others. What we write in the journal should be what we feel at the moment of writing. We need not edit it for others, nor need we worry about careless errors in our writing.

Most importantly, we must be honest with ourselves. This is one time we do not need to create an impression on someone else. Each day will be a snapshot of what we are thinking, what we are feeling, and what we are hoping for ourselves and our future. The tone may change from day to day because our feelings may change. As we read our entries of a month ago, we will begin to see how changes take place in our feelings and outlook. We will understand that the relentless pain we are experiencing at the moment will not be with us forever because we will have a record of times when it was not there, but we also know that as human beings, we will always be susceptible to feelings of pain. This is the beginning of our distancing ourselves from our pain.

Our inner self or our inner voice will begin to emerge as the writing continues. We must try not to be critical of what we write. That critic within us is one of the voices we are trying to still. When those negative, critical ideas begin, we must find a way to ignore them. I do not mean, here, that we will not write about feelings or situations that are painful. Such feelings have an important place in our journal. What does not have a place is the kind of thinking which says *This is useless! You will never be able to change! What do you think you are proving when you do this?* Such voices as these are the ones we must put behind us.

One way to put these voices behind us is to discover where they come from. We begin our journey with a set of topics which will help us find the source of those voices and sketch an outline of who we are.

Journal
Topic One

"I am what I believe...These are my beliefs"

We begin our journal by listing our beliefs about ourselves. Under each belief, we try to explain how we arrived at that belief. If possible, we should try to include details that illustrate that belief. Here are some examples:

> *I believe that I am responsible for the welfare of my family. As the eldest of five children, I was always responsible for their care. My parents always praised me when I sacrificed my own enjoyment to take care of the children. I now get my enjoyment from looking after my family.*

> *I believe that I am not worth anything unless I make more money than my brothers. My brothers and I always competed in sports and games and they always seemed to win. They made me feel I was worthless. The one thing I could do better than they was to earn more money. Now they have to admit that I am worth something when they see my house and car.*

Try to develop four or five of these that seem to describe your belief system. There are no true or untrue answers in this exercise. We write what comes into our head. If we *believe* it is true, that is enough. As we will see, we will be looking at whether we want to change some of these beliefs as well. Later, we may decide that there are other important beliefs which we have omitted. We need not add them to this page. We simply add them to the journal page on the day we think of them. Each journal page represents how we think today.

```
┌─────────────────────────────────┐
│                                 │
│            Journal              │
│          Topic Two              │
│                                 │
└─────────────────────────────────┘
```

"I change who I am when I change my beliefs"

After we have listed our beliefs, we think about them and decide whether they are beliefs that we need to continue to hold. Are they helping to move us in the direction we want to go? If so, we should retain them. If these beliefs are forcing us to live a life that is making us unhappy, we should consider what we can do to change them. Again, we don't have to work out the details here. We just have to express our intention. Here is an example:

My belief about the importance of money is forcing me to do things which prevent me from doing things I think I would like to do. Because money seems to be so important to me, I am working at a job that takes so much time that I don't have time to be with my family. My children are growing up without me.

We need not spend a great deal of time on any of these ideas. As we continue in this process, we will discover that the fleeting, impulsive thought may have a depth that no amount of later analysis can provide. We note our immediate impressions and depend on time and later impressions to strengthen or eliminate them.

```
Journal
Topic Three
```

"My beliefs about my pain strengthen the nature of that pain...These are my beliefs about my pain..."

In this section, we confront our pain. Before listing the beliefs, it might be useful to provide a brief summary of the source of the pain, when it began, what were the circumstances, what was happening in our lives at that time and how we felt about the pain. When that is completed, we list the beliefs we have about the pain and, after each one, describe how we have arrived at that belief. Here are some examples of beliefs about pain:

> *I believe that it is unlikely that anything can be done about this pain because I have been to several doctors, and they cannot find the source of the pain.* *If the doctors cannot find the reason for the pain, how is it possible to provide a cure? I am usually unlucky in life so this is just one more example.*

> *I believe that if I can find the right doctor, he can stop this pain.* *I have always been able to find someone to help me solve problems in my life. Why should this be any different?*

Writing these ideas down usually makes us see our beliefs about our pain in a new way. Again, we need not spend a great deal of time on thinking about this nor discard fleeting ideas as unworthy. We enter them in the journal and see what happens.

Journal
Topic Four

"Some of my beliefs about my pain are not helpful in a healing program... These are the beliefs I would like to change."

As we review our beliefs, we may discover that we are limiting our possibilities by the way we view our pain. If this is the case, we list here those beliefs we wish to change. If there are new beliefs that occur to us, we can add them also. What we are doing here is creating an intention to change. This will provide a direction toward which our inner voice will guide us. Here is a suggested change for one of the beliefs listed above:

> *Just because the doctors have not been able to find the source of my pain is no reason to believe that I will not find it. My new belief will be that when I learn to understand my pain, I will be able to find a way to reduce it.*

> # Journal
> # Topic Five

"Pain affects my life in some important ways"

Here, we list, briefly, the obvious ways that pain has affected our life. We begin with the negative influences it has on our relationships, our jobs, our feelings about ourselves, our future.

Next we list the positive influences our pain has had on the same set of topics. These may seem less obvious at first, but we need to simply allow the ideas to surface. For example, our pain may have limited the way we can socialize with our friends but, on the positive side, it may have provided an opportunity for friends to show they care for us in a way that we have not experienced before.

Journal
Topic Six

"There are other ideas about pain that may apply to me"

In this section we answer any of the following questions by simply responding with the first ideas which come to us. We are not critical, nor do we censor our ideas. For the moment, we let our inner voice respond to these questions:

Are there patterns of pain in my past experience?

Is there an emotional component underlying my pain?

Is there an uncomfortable circumstance that my pain has saved me from?

Is pain part of my identity?

How does my pain involve others?

Are there parts of myself that I am hiding from others? Are these parts related to my pain?

```
┌─────────────────────────────┐
│          Journal            │
│       Topic Seven           │
│                             │
└─────────────────────────────┘
```

"I can imagine a future in which I am free of chronic pain"

In this section, we write a few paragraphs about what our life will be like when we resolve our issues with pain. What challenges can we take on? What dreams can we fulfill? In this way, we are forming a future that is pain free.

```
┌─────────────────────────────┐
│          Journal            │
│       Topic Eight           │
│                             │
└─────────────────────────────┘
```

"There are factors in my job and at home that are obstructing my healing process"

In this section we list those aspects of our life that are creating both physical and emotional stress and, thus, have a negative impact on our healing. It is important to list these things, even though there seems to be nothing to be done about them at this time. We must always keep in mind the fact that change continues whether we notice it or not. Possibilities become realities.

Journal
Topic Nine

"I will become acquainted with my pain"

If you could have a conversation with your pain, what would it tell you?

Write a dialogue between you and your pain. Describe your feelings toward your pain and what your pain needs to tell you.

Allow your intuition and imagination to take over!

Journal
Topic Ten

"My Plan for Healing must include..."

1. The areas of my body in which pain must be reduced.

2. Any belief systems which I may need to change.

3. Those circumstances in my life that must be changed to allow my healing to take place.

4. Those aspects of my future which will change when I resolve my issues with pain.

This concludes the beginning entries in the journal. It may take more than one session to complete this part of the journal. When it is completed, we need only spend fifteen minutes to half an hour with journal entries each day.

Suggestions for Daily Journal Entries

Again, we can enter any ideas we wish in the journal but answering the following questions may help us keep a focus on our exploration.

1. How would I describe my experience of pain today? Minor? Major? Excruciating? No Change?

2. What situations developed today that I felt good about?

3. What situations developed that seemed to make my pain worse? What happened that seemed to reduce my pain?

4. What did I do today to try to further my exploration of healing my pain?

5. What plans do I have for tomorrow to further my healing exploration?

*6. What new insights did I have today that
seem important to understanding myself, my life,
and/or my pain?*

This journal becomes a road to self analysis. I cannot
predict for you where it will lead. Each of us is unique and
we all make our own exciting discoveries. As we continue,
we will gain more and more confidence in responding to our
inner voice. It may be the guide that we will come to depend
on as we make our choices in our healing program.

The next chapters will provide exercises which will help
with this exploration. In each case, we can allow our inner
voice or intuition to help us select those activities which will
help us. The journal is only the first step, but our self-analysis
has begun.

- 8 -

Healing Exercises

Once we have developed some ideas in our journal about the nature of our pain, we are ready to explore other possibilities for our healing. The following pages provide exercises which may be helpful. As we read through the possibilities, we should allow our intuition to play a major part in the selection of appropriate therapies.

The following exercises promote a sense of well-being and empowerment and expand the individual consciousness. These exercises are not new. Their origin dates back well over 5000 years to ancient civilizations of both East and West. They serve as the foundation for our healing process and they provide the strength to release distorted energy patterns.

We begin by focusing on the way we breathe. The essence of life comes through our breath. As infants, we breathe with the diaphragm. Our abdomen expands with the inhalation and contracts with exhalation. But somewhere in life, we lose this efficient manner of breathing and, to regain it as adults, we need to become aware of the function of the diaphragm in breathing.

Breathing with the chest is associated with high stress situations. It is known as the *fight or flight response* which causes the body to go into a survival mode. This stressful state is valuable only in brief moments of danger when large amounts of oxygen are needed in a short period of time. When we maintain this mode on a daily basis, it becomes destructive and depletes our body of its energy. More importantly, it can intensify the experience of pain.

These exercises help us to develop an understanding of the relationship between our body and our emotions. As our body relaxes, it begins to release the negative emotions which it has repressed. These emotions then rise to our conscious awareness. We also gain an intuitive insight into how the blocked energy patterns distort the body's natural healing process. Experiment with these exercises and rely on your intuition to select those which are most beneficial.

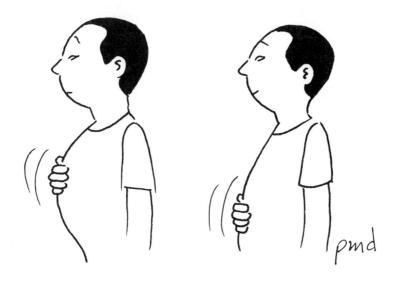

Chest Breathing   **Diaphragmatic Breathing**

Place one hand on your abdomen and one on your chest. If you are breathing from your diaphragm, the hand placed on the abdomen will rise and fall with each inhalation and exhalation, and there will be little or no movement with the hand on the chest. If the hand on the chest is the one which is moving, then you are breathing from the chest.

DIAPHRAGMATIC BREATHING

◆ *Assume a comfortable position.*

◆ *Begin to inhale and exhale through your nostrils. If you have difficulty breathing through the nostrils, then breathe through the mouth.*

◆ *When you inhale, imagine that your breath is flowing down to the pelvic region.*

◆ *Become aware of how the abdomen rises with the inhalation and gently drops inward with exhalation.*

◆ *You may become aware of some unevenness in your breathing. Simply allow the breath to flow without force.*

◆ *As you perform this exercise, become aware of any decrease in respiration, heart rate, blood pressure, muscle tension, and pain. See yourself inhaling oxygen and energy.*

◆ *Continue this exercise for three to five minutes.*

The healthy blood flow and increased endorphin production resulting from this exercise will develop an enhanced sense of well-being.

An added benefit for many people in these exercises is that they connect to the feelings which may have been obscured through the body's effort to protect itself from the harmful effects of those emotions.

The way the body protects itself from hurt is through various defense mechanisms that freeze the diaphragm. By freezing the diaphragm and shifting the breathing to the chest, an individual soon learns to cover up unwanted feelings, thoughts, and desires.

It is not uncommon to re-experience trauma that has appeared to have been tucked safely away. As the mind and body relaxes, it begins to release unhealthy memories which rise to the surface of the conscious mind. Often these experiences are so disturbing that health clinicians prescribe medications which help to curb these negative thought patterns and allow the individual to function better in society. Such medications may be useful in maintaining a normal daily life. Nevertheless, these disturbing thoughts and emotional patterns are being held under the surface below the conscious awareness of the individual where they continue to retard the healing process. It is the acknowledgment and release of these thought patterns that allow us to move confidently toward our healing.

GENERAL RELAXATION

This exercise is the foundation that will help reduce stress and anxiety and enhance a sense of well-being. It will be beneficial to audio-tape this exercise.

◆ *Bring your awareness to your breath. Notice the coolness in your nostrils when you inhale and the warmth when you exhale.*

◆ *Just observe the breath without trying to control or force it. Just let it flow easily and naturally in whatever way is most comfortable for you.*

◆ *Become aware of the steady rise and fall of your abdomen. It rises with the inhalation and falls with exhalation.*

◆ *Feel a coolness with the inhalation and warmth with the exhalation.*

◆ *Bring your awareness to your forehead, your eyes and eyebrows, cheeks and jaws, and the corners of your mouth. Relax your tongue.*

◆ *Let that awareness move downward into the neck and shoulder muscles.*

◆ *Relax your upper arms, elbows, lower arms, wrists, fingers, and finger tips.*

◆ *Now with your awareness, let the relaxation return upward through the finger tips, wrists, lower arms, upper arms, and shoulders.*

◆ *Relax the neck and chest muscles.*

◆ *Bring your awareness to the internal organs.*

◆ *Now let the awareness move downward to the pelvic region.*

◆ *Relax the thighs, knees, calves, ankles, feet, and toes.*

◆ *Now let that relaxation return up through the toes, the soles of the feet, the ankles, and heels.*

◆ *Relax the calves, knees, and thighs.*

◆ *Bring your awareness to the pelvic region and the base of the spine.*

◆ *Relax the muscles up the back, one vertebra at a time, all the way up to the neck.*

◆ *Relax the muscles in the face, the cheeks, the jaws, and the corners of the mouth.*

◆ *Relax the muscles in the forehead, eyes, and eyebrows.*

◆ *Relax the scalp.*

◆ *Let your body be completely relaxed from the top of your head down to your feet.*

◆ *To receive the benefits from this exercise, remain in this position as long as you are comfortable.*

Passive and Dominant Nostril Patterns

Eastern philosophers have long believed in the importance of the breath in enhancing the flow of the body's energy. Most of us are not aware that every two or three hours the breath in one nostril flows more easily than the other. The nostril that is flowing more freely is called the dominant nostril. The opposite nostril is called the passive nostril. You may discover your own nostril dominance by blocking one nostril and comparing the ease in which the breath flows through the other.

Between these cycles there is a period of time when breath flows equally through both nostrils. The ancient Indian philosophers called this the wedding of the right and left nostrils or equal night and equal day. This equal balance of breath also occurs at higher levels of awareness, such as the moment of orgasm, or profound meditation.

The readiness for certain activities is influenced by this nostril dominance. The right nostril dominance indicates sympathetic arousal. When it is open, one is ready for such physical activity as eating, playing, and working. The left nostril dominance indicates parasympathetic activity such as sleeping, reading, and listening.

Sometimes when the body chemistry is not in balance, the nostrils do not change. In these cases it would be wise to select activities which are appropriate to the dominant nostril. For example, if the left nostril is dominant you may not be as successful in physical activity as in passive activity. It is valuable to experiment with the influence of nostril dominance on your own activities.

Following are some techniques which you may use to change nostril dominance:

◆ *Lie on the side opposite of the nostril you want to open. Breathe diaphragmatically for two to five minutes or until open.*

◆ *Focus your awareness on the nostril desired to be open. Feel the breath flow in and out of the nostril until it opens. With practice, you can change the flow of breath in the nostrils at will.*

◆ *Close one nostril with your fingers, cotton, or gauze until the opposite opens.*

Alternate Nostril Breathing

The primary benefit of this exercise is the soothing effect it has on emotions. Try to perform this exercise one to three times daily to maintain emotional balance.

Although there are several methods of alternate nostril breathing one simple method is described here.

♦ *First determine which nostril is dominant. Do this by blocking one nostril at a time and breathing in and out of it to determine which nostril is flowing more freely. This will be your dominant nostril.*

♦ *Block the passive nostril with either a finger or thumb. Exhale and inhale through the dominant nostril three times.*

♦ *Then block the dominant nostril and exhale and inhale through the passive nostril three times.*

This constitutes one cycle. Repeat this cycle two more times until you have completed three cycles.

Progressive Relaxation

We often retain stress and pain in our muscles. The following exercise can aid in the release of that stress. In performing this exercise, try to become aware of the parts of your body that have been blocked by the distorted patterns of stress or emotion. As you do the exercise, try to sense the release of the toxins that are stored in the muscle tissue. This exercise is easily performed if it has been audio-taped in advance.

This exercise can be done sitting, or lying down. It involves contracting, holding, and releasing muscle groups. In the muscle contractions, it is important to observe one's capacity and not try to go beyond it. As you perform the exercise observe your feelings and emotions. It is important to breathe diaphragmatically and not to hold the breath.

◆ *Become aware of the flow of the breath as it flows in and out of the nostrils.*

◆ *Bring your awareness to the facial muscles. Inhale, slowly tightening the forehead and the cheeks. Tighten the face like a prune.*

◆ *Exhale and gently release the muscles. Take a few slow, even breaths and repeat, slowly, two more times.*

◆ *Inhale. Make a fist with both hands and tighten all the muscles up the arms to the chest and hold.*

◆ *Exhale and release the muscles.*

◆ *Repeat, slowly, two more times.*

◆ *Inhale, and gently tighten the abdomen. Hold as long as comfortable.*

◆ *Exhale and release.*

◆ *Repeat this procedure two more times.*

◆ *Inhale and extend your heels away from your body and point your toes toward your head.*

◆ *Tighten the muscles up your legs to the buttocks and hold.*

◆ *Exhale, release.*

◆ *Repeat this procedure two more times.*

◆ *On the next inhalation, tighten all the muscles from the feet to the top of the head. The feet, the ankles, the calves, the thighs, the buttocks. Tighten the abdomen.*

◆ *Make a fist with the hands and tighten the arms up the shoulders to the chest muscles.*

◆ *Tighten all the muscles in your face, forehead, cheeks, jaws, and mouth. Hold.*

◆ *Slowly release all the muscles.*

◆ *Repeat this procedure two more times.*

◆ *Allow yourself time to sense this state of deep relaxation and, when you are ready, open your eyes.*

Emptying the Mind of Unwanted Thoughts

Our minds are in constant activity. Minor impressions and major thoughts pursue each other endlessly. Some of these thoughts are detrimental to our healing. We need to find a way to neutralize them. This exercise is intended to provide a method of emptying the mind of these unwanted thoughts. With practice you will come to know that your thoughts have no hold or power over you if you don't identify with them. These thoughts just dissipate on their own because you don't give them any energy. They slowly fade and die. Eventually they no longer bother you. You will come to see that they are just old worn out tapes which no longer have any influence over you.

Practice this exercise one to five minutes. Extend the time as you feel able.

- *Bring your complete awareness to the breath. Just become a witness. Don't force or try to control it. Just let it flow in a way which is easy and natural for you.*

- *Feel the coolness in your nostrils when you inhale and the warmth when you exhale.*

- *Notice the steady rise and fall of your abdomen with each breath.*

- *If your mind wanders, just bring it back to the breath. Continue to watch the flow of the breath.*

Your goal is to experience longer periods of time in which you are not connected to the thought flow. Just focus on the breath.

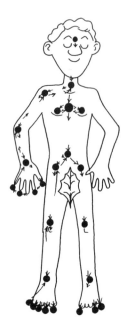

Sixty-One Points

This exercise helps to reach a very deep level of relaxation and to revitalize the mind and the body. It is said to equal two hours of deep sleep. As you perform the exercise, try to tune into specific parts of the body and detect any imbalance in the system.

In this exercise you will bring your awareness to specific points in the body. You may choose to visualize a color or a shape, or you may select a sound, or in some way bring your awareness to these points. It would be well to audio-tape this exercise.

Bring your awareness to the following points:

◆ *The space between the two eyebrows.*

◆ *The throat region.*

◆ *The right shoulder joint, the right elbow joint, the right wrist joint.*

◆ *The tip of the right thumb, the tip of the right index finger, the tip of the right middle finger, the tip of the right ring finger, the tip of the right baby finger.*

◆ *Return to the right wrist joint, the right elbow joint, the right shoulder joint, to the throat center.*

◆ *The left shoulder joint, the left elbow joint, the left wrist joint.*

◆ *The tip of the left thumb, the tip of the left index finger, the tip of the left middle finger, the tip of the left ring finger, and the tip of the left baby finger.*

◆ *The left wrist joint, the left elbow joint, the left shoulder joint, to the throat center.*

◆ *The heart center (the space between the two breasts).*

◆ *The right nipple, back to the heart center.*

◆ *The left nipple, back to the heart center.*

◆ *The navel center.*

- *The right hip joint, to the right knee joint, to the right ankle joint.*

- *The tip of the right big toe, the tip of the right second toe, the tip of the right middle toe, the tip of the right fourth toe, the tip of the right baby toe.*

- *Back to the right ankle joint, to the right knee-joint, to the right hip joint.*

- *Back to the navel center.*

- *The left hip joint, to the left knee joint, to the left ankle joint.*

- *The tip of the left big toe, the tip of the left second toe, the tip of the left middle toe, the tip of the left fourth toe, the tip of the left baby toe.*

- *Back to the left ankle joint, to the left knee joint, to the left hip joint.*

- *Back to the navel center.*

- *To the heart center.*

- *The throat center.*

◆ *The space between the two eyebrows.*

◆ *Try to maintain this deep sense of relaxation for an extended period of time. When you are ready, return to a normal level of consciousness.*

Spinal Breath

Imagine a current of vital energy in your body which moves up and down your spine. Think of this energy as the life force of the body. As you perform this exercise, it will help to restore a healthy flow of energy up and down the spinal cord.

◆ *As you exhale, visualize a current of energy flowing down to the base of the spine, and without any pauses, inhale, and allow the vital force to flow upward to the crown of the head.*

◆ *Repeat this breathing process and imagine a light or a wave flowing up and down the spine.*

Take time to develop an awareness of this life force flowing in your body.

Sleep Induction

Many people experience insomnia due to the mental and physical stress which complicates their healing. Developing the ability to sleep is a very empowering achievement.

The first step in this process is to neutralize the issues that are bothering you. If there are issues that you can't resolve, you can put them to rest by firmly deciding that you will deal with them on the following day. Let that be enough. Do not dwell on the possibilities at this time. Firmness with yourself is important.

Turn your attention now to your physical state. When you go to bed you will follow a series of positions which the body does naturally but which are interrupted by stress and pain.

◆ *Lie on your left side.*

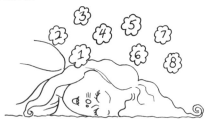

◆ *Inhale and exhale 8 times, this opens the right nostril.*

◆ *Lie on the right side and inhale and exhale 16 times, this opens the left nostril.*

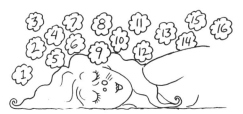

◆ *Then lie on your back and inhale and exhale 32 times.*

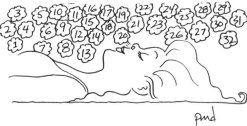

◆ *Those individuals who are unable to assume these positions because of physical limitations may perform this exercise in the following manner.*

◆ *Bring your mental awareness to the right nostril and inhale and exhale slowly from the diaphragm 8 times.*

◆ *Then focus the breath on the left nostril and inhale and exhale 16 times.*

◆ *Bring your awareness to the space between the two nostrils and inhale and exhale 32 times.*

Eventually the number of inhalations and exhalations required to reach the sleep state can be reduced to ten each cycle. Soon you will learn to go to sleep in a matter of seconds. If you find that you have no problem going to sleep but wake up off and on because of discomfort, then just repeat the exercise and you will gently fall back to sleep.

VISUALIZATION

One of the most important aspects of healing is a sense of serenity which will allow the body to heal. Often we are unable to obtain this in our day to day existence so we must set aside a time to create that sense for ourselves in order to let the body heal. The following visualization is a good way to lead yourself into a period of serenity. Perform this exercise in a place that is free of interruptions. Audio-Tape the visualization and allow yourself time to experience its effects.

Imagine yourself walking in a meadow, where an enchanted forest emerges in front of you.

You notice a path leading into the forest, and it welcomes you. As you enter the forest, you immediately sense the peace, tranquillity, and safety of this sacred place.

The trees are tall, their branches reaching towards the sunlight high above. The light filters down through the green of the trees, creating a dappled carpet of light on the forest floor.

A soft breeze whispers through the branches and leaves, caressing your body.

The spirits of the breeze have messages that speak to your soul.

Your body responds to the soft light, to the breezes, to the sounds of the birds and creatures of the forest, welcoming you.

Ahead, you see a clearing with a fallen log and a place that seems to have been created for you to rest upon. Sit here and experience your connection to the earth.

All of the worries, concerns, and tension in your body begin to leave you. You feel centered, grounded, and at peace. The energy of the forest moves through you, connecting you to the earth. You are at peace.

Composed by

Kate Brennan Anderson

GROUNDING

Grounding allows us to create strong boundaries. That is, we become aware of our own power and our own body. It provides us with a healthy space and strength. With the breathing and relaxation exercises, it is the foundation of this work. It allows us to be in the present moment. We are not caught up in the shadows of the past or the anxiety of the future. We become grounded through the earth's energy.

This exercise can be performed standing, sitting, or lying down. Focusing the awareness can be done through visualizing an image, hearing a sound, or feeling a sensation. In the exercise, use any of these techniques to focus your awareness.

◆ *Allow the breath to flow down to the lowest part of your abdomen. Focus your awareness just above the pubic bone.*

◆ *Project that energy all the way to the floor. Send the energy into the ground as deep as you can go.*

◆ *Using your imagination, allow your feet to grow roots as if they are extending into the ground.*

◆ *Allow gravity to pull your feet down and feel the weight of your feet on the floor. Now feel the energy and weight of the floor supporting your feet.*

◆ *Allow that energy to flow deep into the ground. Now feel the energy to flow back up though the ground into the soles of the feet.*

◆ *Feel the returning energy flowing throughout the body.*

When you are grounded, you may experience any or all of these feelings: Your body will feel very heavy. You may feel tingling sensations from your legs down into your feet. You may feel energy rising up from the ground into the feet. You will feel a sense of power and vitality. You will feel a strong connection to those around you.

The exercises in this chapter are doorways to a deeper understanding of that inner self that is hidden, so often, by worries, fears, and anger. Each of us finds that self in our own way, but the soft meditative quality of these exercises can allow us a gradual internal discovery that, sometimes, cannot be put into words. Experiment with them and make your own discoveries!

- 9 -

The Healing Transition

As we continue with our journal and exercises, we will begin to develop a clearer idea of those therapies that we can incorporate into our healing program. The transition from inner analysis to a reaching out for the alternative healing techniques begins here.

If we are concerned with the problems of suppressed emotional trauma, for example, we need to pay particular attention to ways which we can uncover and release those buried feelings. This is not simple. We may have a sense within ourselves that there is something troubling us but which we cannot identify. One way to retrieve these memories is through the use of the journal procedures discussed earlier. The meditative exercises discussed in the last chapter have also proven to be an excellent way to open those closed doors. However, these may not be sufficient to uncover years of suppressed anger or emotion. If this is the case, we have available to us a number of professionals who can support us in this effort.

There are three ways which these memories can be retrieved through the help of a professional. The most common method is through the help of a psychotherapist. In general, this procedure depends on "talking through" the issues. The techniques vary widely and they can be very effective. A second method of retrieval of these memories is through the use of hypnotherapy. Many psychotherapists are also trained in this technique but there are other certified hypnotherapists who can be of help as well. This procedure leads the client into a slightly altered state in which the subconscious mind is allowed to surface bringing with it these memories.

A cautionary note: In recent years, there has been some concern about both psychotherapists and hypnotherapists "suggesting" memories. A competent therapist will take measures to be sure this does not happen. If you are in any way concerned about this, feel free to ask the therapist what measures he or she takes to avoid this problem.

An increasingly common alternative for retrieving these memories is through the use of Mind/Body techniques. In these procedures, the therapist uses techniques to manipulate body energy in ways which seem to retrieve these traumatic memories. In my own practice, this is a very common occurrence. Some clients have been very successful in releasing suppressed traumas.

But whatever method you select, only you can evaluate how effective it is in meeting your needs. If, after a reasonable amount of time, you seem not to be making progress, begin looking at other possibilities. It may be that you are ready for another type of therapy.

In addition to emotional trauma, there are other aspects of chronic pain which we also need to work on. There are many alternative methods which may complement the treatments we are presently receiving and which might be very helpful in our healing process. As we explore the different treatments mentioned in this chapter, we must always be clear about how the method is expected to bring about our healing. Professionals in any of these fields will be glad to provide a description of how the method works on our body.

Alternative Healing Methods

For convenience sake, these alternative approaches to healing are divided into eight different categories. It is important to understand that this is only a summary of the available possibilities.

As we begin this search, we must remember that ultimately, we are each in charge of our own healing process and the methods and the individual(s) that work with us are there only to assist, coach, and provide a safe environment. If, in any way, we feel uncomfortable with a treatment or team of therapists, we should find someone we feel more comfortable with and that we trust. We should be aware, too, that many of these treatments are not reimbursable from insurance companies, so the costs and methods of payment must be clearly worked out before treatment begins.

AROMATHERAPY is any therapy that uses scents which are absorbed by the cells of the skin, inhaled through the nostrils, and used to treat emotional disorders and promote a sense of well-being. Examples are herbal scents and flower essences.

BODY WORK manipulates muscles, bones, and, tendons to bring them into proper alignment. This increases the energy flow and the release of toxins, thus allowing the body to heal itself. Examples are Massage Therapy, Chiropractic Care, Osteopathic Therapy, Physical Therapy, CranioSacral therapy, and Rolphing.

ENERGY THERAPY is any therapy that restores the natural flow of energy to the body by opening up blocked energy channels. Examples are Acupressure, Acupuncture, and such hands on healing techniques as Reiki, Mari El, Energy Chelation, and Vibrational Toning.

MEDICINE is any therapy that uses medications to attempt to treat symptoms or alleviate them. In addition to allopathic medicine, they include homeopathic therapy, herbal therapy, Bach flower remedies, and ayurvedic medicines.

NUTRITIONAL THERAPY is any therapy that uses nutrition as a means of healing the body such as the macrobiotic diets, vegetarianism, and other nutritional regimens.

PSYCHOTHERAPY is any therapy that uses psychological analysis to help understand underlying emotional issues that may contribute to disease, pain, or stress. These techniques may include psychoanalysis, counseling, and clinical hypnosis.

RELAXATION THERAPY is any therapy that incorporates breathing, visualization, and music techniques to induce a state of relaxation. This promotes the general free flow of energy, reduces stress, and strengthens the nervous system. These methods may include Rebirthing, Rogian therapy, and Yoga breathing techniques.

OTHER TYPES OF HEALING METHODS are healing through prayer, spiritual healing, bio-energetics, core-energetics, shamanism, and oxygen therapy.

Most therapists will use more than one of these techniques in their practice. When a typical client comes to me, I discuss the various techniques and modalities that can be incorporated in their healing process. Together, we decide what would be the appropriate therapy. It is not unusual to explore several possibilities in the course of treatments. These explorations are based on the feedback that the clients give me about their response to the treatments.

When we are working with a therapist, one of the most valuable things we can do is provide feedback about the effectiveness of the treatment as we go. If a treatment is not effective, the therapist needs that information to adjust the technique if necessary. It is possible that a particular type of treatment simply is not appropriate for an individual. If that is the case, there is little point in wasting the time of the client or the therapist.

As we search for people to assist us in our healing, it is wise to keep in mind that in every profession, there are charlatans. They are not as widespread as some would like us to believe, but they are there. Most healing professionals take their responsbilities seriously and being effective is important to them. If, however, you begin to feel that a therapist has another agenda, lose no time in finding another therapist. Not only will your money be wasted if you remain with such a therapist, but the negative emotions which build up in such a relationship can be detrimental to your health. Again, if you have begun to be guided by the inner voice through your journal writing, you will have little difficulty in knowing when something is wrong for you.

Creating a Healing Environment

Another consideration in our healing program is our surrounding environment. The following elements are important influences on the process of our healing. We may have already identified one or more of them in our journal as we began our self-analysis. These elements are reviewed only briefly here, as the focus of this book is not on these issues. Nevertheless, each of these influences plays a major role in the healing process. Again, intuitional insights can be of great help. In addition, there are counselors and consultants in each of these areas which can assist us in thinking through our needs.

RELATIONSHIPS: The many relationships in our life can be comforting, supportive, and loving, but they can also be harmful, abusive, or inhibiting. In each case they have an important influence on our healing process. As we begin our healing plan, we should analyze the important relationships in our life and the ways in which they are helpful or detrimental to the process. Are we in relationships which usually leave us feeling depressed or inadequate? If so, what can be done about the situation? Do we have relationships which seem to provide us strength and courage? Are we making the most of these benefits? Understanding the effects of these relationships can be the beginning of healthy change.

JOBS AND CAREER GOALS: Our jobs or careers often create difficulties in implementing our healing plan because they are sources of stress and pressure. We can easily feel inadequate to the demands of our work even though we may, in fact, be performing acceptably. We may have already identified challenges in this area in our journal. Our healing plan must provide solutions to these challenges, whether they are alternative job or career choices or a changed attitude about the importance of this aspect of our life.

FINANCES: Worries over finances are a part of everyone's existence, but they become particularly difficult in the experience of chronic pain. It is important to confront these issues and make the best decisions possible under the circumstances, so that we can go on with our healing process. What is very important is that we not continue in the same destructive pattern which brought us to our present state.

A frequent source of anger is brought about by the additional burdens of the treatment of pain. The legal, medical, and insurance issues must be confronted and resolved so that the frustration will not interfere with our recovery process.

RECREATION: A part of our healing plan must allow for periods of play, enjoyment, and laughter. These are necessary to keep the healthy perspective we are working for, as well as the benefits of reduced stress and the increased endorphin production which contribute to the reduction of pain. Recreation should be scheduled in our lives as regularly as therapy.

SPIRITUAL PURSUITS: Spirituality, in this context, is defined by each individual, but it refers to any activity which brings us an awareness of reality that transcends our ordinary, daily activities. For some people this is a church activity, for others it is immersion in music or the arts, and for still others, it is their connection with nature. As we pursue breathing and meditating exercises we will develop an enriched sense of spiritual experiences. Attention to these experiences will enhance the quality of our healing process.

Transition to Health

Following is a page from a journal of a chronic pain client. It seems to summarize the gamut of emotions in dealing with chronic pain. It is included here as an example of the work in progress. At some point, we must begin to make a transition to a state of health. This transition requires changes in both the body and the mind.

A Safe Place

I am being bombarded within and outside of my body. Hurt, memories, problems... my mind cannot rest.

My head hurts. I feel sick, angry, alone. When I look inside my mind toward my pain, everything around me is black and still... empty... lifeless... No stars or planets, just cold, dead space.

Except a blinding, raging, swirling red entity that is trying to annihilate me. All of my life, for as long as I can remember, it has been my constant and unwelcome companion.

Why has it chosen me? Why do I allow it to constantly disrupt my life?

I am trying to remember....I will think of what I've been told by those who are the experts with pain.

"Go into your pain, look at it. What color is it? Don't fight it, that only makes it stronger. You can't control it that way. Embrace the pain. Hold it. Go into it." It is me.

I will find a safe place... Somewhere I will find refuge... a sanctuary. I'm trying slow, deep breaths. I am aware of my breathing. The pain is there. I acknowledge it, and leave it to continue breathing... taking slow, deep breaths.

I see streaks of color here and there. My body feels so light, so free, almost airy. I hear birds singing and the sound of water... the ocean!

Now I see the blue sky full of clouds and rainbows. Pastel colors everywhere. Below me is a beautiful, quiet garden. A safe place. It is full of birds, butterflies and animals... all peaceful and content. And flowers... they are gorgeous and they are everywhere!

I see a lovely stream flowing gently down to a little pond. It then flows on into a beautiful waterfall. I love the sounds of the water, the ocean... it fills me with contentment.

I feel my breath, warm and gentle going into and through my body, then cool and soothing as it leaves me. I feel serene and awed by such beauty that can only be touched by God. No red or black remains to mar this scene.

When I look up, there is a majestic mountain range... snow-capped...surrounded by clouds and mists. It almost reaches the rainbow. From very, very far away I hear the melody of a harp.

This pain, I can finally see, is me. It is what I do to myself when I allow the outside to intrude on my serenity.

I will set boundaries. Problems, worries, yes, they are there. I will act upon or change what I can and let the rest go. They are already irrelevant... They are part of my past with no power over me. They are just worries, not facts.

I will go to my "Safe Place." My mind and body are whole.

I am at peace with my mind and myself.

A New Journey Begins

Whether we have selected one of the several therapies in this book or whether we are part of a treatment clinic, there will come a time when we will make the transition from therapy to a concern for maintaining a state of wellness.

This is a time to remember that chronic pain is not an individual matter. It affects everyone who is connected to us. A spouse or child may also be exhausted by the worry over our condition or have come to feel that there must be an end to their sacrifice. These are difficult problems to confront and if our healing is to continue to grow, we must find ways to understand and accept those feelings without sacrificing ourself in the process.

We should keep in mind that guilt is an easy emotion to manifest, but it is damaging to the health of everyone involved. We should try to avoid placing or accepting blame for any of the circumstances in which we find ourself. We need to focus on the those things which will help us heal.

From time to time, there are those aspects of our living situation which are detrimental to our healing. We must find the strength to eliminate them if we are to continue on our path. If we are honest with ourselves and others we will find creative ways in which to resolve these situations. In any case, we cannot allow the forces which created our dilemma to interfere with our healing.

Our transition to health is complete when we stop thinking of these activities as *healing* activities and begin to refer to them as *wellness* activities. Our identity will no longer include the chronic pain label. We will have found a different way of thinking about ourselves.

For information on seminars or
audio-tapes, contact:

New Energy Press
1225 LaSalle, Suite 1604
Minneapolis, MN 55403

INDEX